# NO ONE PREPARED
# ME FOR THIS

To Linda -
Best Wishes
from
Kathleen Nielson
Oct 4, 1989

*After great pain a formal feeling comes—*
*The Nerves sit ceremonious, like Tombs—*
*The stiff Heart questions was it He, that bore,*
*And Yesterday, or Centuries before?*

*The Feet, mechanical, go round—*
*Of Ground, or Air, or Ought—*
*A wooden way*
*Regardless grown,*
*A Quartz contentment, like a stone—*

*This is the Hour of Lead—*
*Remembered, if outlived,*
*As Freezing persons, recollect the Snow—*
*First—Chill—then Stupor—then the letting go.*

*Emily Dickinson*

# No One Prepared Me For This

Kathleen V. Nielson

Intermountain Health Care
Home Health Agency
Salt Lake City

The IHC Hospice program supports the philosophy of providing care to people whose circumstances are similar to those of the author of this book.

*I dedicate this book to you, the reader.
It is my hope that from its content you will
glean some thoughts that lead you to a
deeper understanding of the trauma
of living with illness and death, and that
possibly you might see some positive action
to use in your own life as you come
to deal with the illness and death
of those around you.*

## *Foreword*

While we strive to establish our individuality, it seems equally important to know that we are not alone, that others have had similar experiences. This sense of universality is a valued element in friendship, in psychotherapy, and in literature.

The book you have in your hands is a poignant account of the struggle and loss prompted by the death of a mate. It encompasses the unpredictable and the predictable, the shock, sadness, anger, confusion, and relief that result when death touches us directly.

In sharp, penetrating descriptions, the author opens for us a window into this most inevitable of all experiences. For those who have had death come to someone close, this may sound a familiar echo. For those who have yet to encounter this loss, the book may help us anticipate this experience.

Stuart Drescher, Ph.D.
University of Utah

# Acknowledgments

There are many people to whom I owe thanks for their continued support throughout the writing of this book. A very special thank-you to Helen Rollins, who first came into my life as a Hospice nurse and has remained a dear friend. Her encouragement throughout the writing of this book was a constant motivation. A generous thank-you to Roger Smedley, my financial counselor, who has not only offered sound advice in finance, but has consistently believed in me, often more than I have believed in myself. His confidence in this project has been truly appreciated.

A special thanks to Charlotte and Sondra, who were always willing to listen through tears to the rough drafts of each segment. And to Kate, Brent, Pam, Phil, and Robyn, who upon reading the finished manuscript rendered the praise I needed to confidently seek publication, a heartfelt thanks.

To my dear friend Lola, who for the past thirty years has shared joy and pain with me, and has generously given long-distance telephone time to discuss the progress of this work, thank you. Gratitude is also extended to my brother David, for his unfailing support and encouragement.

A most gracious thank-you to the Hospice organizations that have allowed me the privilege of guest-lecturing for them. There I have been able to read some of my stories and learn that others share my feelings.

To Trudy McMurrin, who has taken me by the hand through the editing and the publication of this book, and has answered all questions with enthusiasm, a grateful thank-you.

I wish to thank my children with all my heart. I hope they have endured this project unscathed. They have been understanding and supportive beyond belief as I have slugged through the turbulence of vividly reliving this emotional experience.

I would also like to acknowledge IHC's Home Health/Hospice division for the support they have given this manuscript. Working with them has been a most rewarding experience.

"We've Only Just Begun"
(Paul Williams / Roger Nichols), Irving Music Inc. BMI

"Bridge Over Troubled Water"
Paul Simon (words and music)

"Blowin' In The Wind"
Bob Dylan, M. Witmark & Sons ASCAP

"The Rose"
Amanda McBroom

"The Sounds of Silence"
Paul Simon, Eclectic Music Co.

## *Introduction*

No one prepared me for this. That's for sure. But then I guess we don't often feel much prepared for what comes our way. How many of us have been prepared for the major emotional events of life? The first real love? The first real heartache? Marriage? Birth? Divorce? Death? No one can really tell us what it's going to be like. And, true enough, life's experiences are different for each one of us. However, we do "grow" through each of these challenges. As least that's what they all tell me. But then most of them are not where I am, or where I've been, and they really don't know.

It just seems to me that somehow it should all be easier. Especially death. Death, and the after-the-death, and the struggle to begin again. Sometimes I just don't get it. We all know it's coming to each of us. It's just around the corner, or down the street. Elusive, but there. No one wants to talk about it. And, sadly enough, after it happens no one wants to talk about it then either. And here are all these people experiencing or witnessing this monumentally humongous, traumatic event, and no one else wants to know about it. So we mourners tend to harbor our grief instead of letting it out. After all, we don't want to make others uncomfortable. And too often, the grief or the pain becomes a tool for us, a crutch, an excuse, or a weapon of guilt to beat ourselves with.

We think we understand it. It's a necessary process. But I think of my aged parents, and I don't want them to die. I really want them to go on and on with me. I suppose they felt the same about their parents.

I have come to the conclusion, however, that it's the finality that is so scary. Someone is in your life and then he's not. Bingo! He's gone but he's not gone, because you keep picking up his tennis racket or you find that long-lost favorite shirt. Sometimes his actual presence can still be felt. That's *really* scary! But it's also comforting, and it's also reassuring.

I will have to admit that above anything else, experiencing the death of my husband has impressed upon me the belief that this ending we meet here, death, as we refer to it, is not a total wipeout. In fact, I'm not so sure that he isn't the lucky one. Don't get me wrong, I'm not campaigning for the trip. I just suppose it's probably not all that bad for the deceased.

But for some reason, and I do believe there's a reason, I am still here plugging away at the bills and the laundry. If indeed it's true that we grow through adversity, I should be ten feet tall by now from all the "growing" I've been doing over the past few years. But I look the same to me. It's true, though, that the inside has changed. Priorities have shifted. It's more important to read to my seven-year-old, and it's more important to listen to my seventeen-year-old. It's more important not to harbor bad feelings, and it's more important to express my love.

You know, someone told me once, and you've probably heard it too, that if we took a pot and everyone put their troubles into it and then it was passed again and we were allowed to draw out only the troubles we wanted, we would all choose our own. What do you think of that? I think I wouldn't want anyone to have to have mine.

I will confess, though, that sharing my troubles, my pain, and my fears, has enabled me to work through them and to go on. I am the luckiest person alive to have the friends I have. They have given me the space and time to tell of my loneliness and of how I fear never being truly loved again. But it's still so difficult, and it seems sometimes as if life is just degrees of difficulty.

Then I meet someone new, or the kids help do the dishes without being asked, and the sun comes out again. It always does. The flowers bloom and the good stuff starts all over again. True, life's never the same, but it can still be great, and it is a natural happening. That's just the way it is.

# No One Prepared Me For This

We are running toward each other along the shore of a lake. Gentle waves are lapping against the rocky shoreline, and each little ripple of water is a silver shimmer of light from the setting sun. It is almost summer and warm. Perspiration holds my pink tee shirt close to my body. I am feeling suspended, as if in slow motion, and I feel the stretch and burn of each muscle as I sprint to close the space between us. I can see him clearly now. His grin is broad and the whiteness of his even teeth exaggerates the slight space between the two in front. His longish blond hair is pulled back by the force of his movement, exposing his widow's peak. He is straining now as I am, and he is clearly winning the race. He is passing the line we are both striving for, but he is still running, still coming toward me, and I am wondering what he will do when we meet. We're almost to touch now, and he is reaching out his hand so that I will know not to go past him. I am slowing my pace so that I can catch his hand, and he has me with both arms. He has grabbed me and lifted me off the ground. We are turning around and around as I see lake and sunset, then trees and mountains, lake and sunset, then trees and mountains. I am slightly dizzy, but he is slowing down and I feel my feet once again precariously placed upon the ground. His embrace feels warm and safe and he's bending down to kiss me. I relax my mouth to receive his soft warm caress and want it to last forever, but somehow the darkness of night has quickly come upon us and we turn reluctantly to the car. The shoreline is rocky and with the fading light it is becoming difficult to find our way. The moist, uneven ground causes us to slip and stumble. We have clasped our hands tightly to help each other as we take turns leading. The car seems farther away than either of us remembered, and I hold on tighter. Suddenly, he has tripped, as if a snare had been set for him, and he slips from my grasp. I can hear him struggling, trying to get up, but I can't see where he's fallen. I catch a glimpse of movement, but it doesn't stay with me and I call out to him. He answers and his voice sounds like a soft echo. I become frightened and I search frantically for him, tripping over sticks, stumbling into the lake's shallow edge. Slipping wildly, I try to free myself from the soft, oozing mud that has encased my shoes and holds me fast. Alone and trembling, I strain to hear even the slightest sounds. Aside from my pounding heart, the only sound is the water gently lapping against the shoreline. A cool breeze rises from the lake and gently rearranges my hair. I hear a rustle as if leaves are stirring and open my eyes to see the nurse attending Dave's I.V. The air conditioner beside me has kicked on and I listen to its droning as the attendant in white smiles, nods, and leaves the room. My nose begins to sting as the tears well over the rim and slowly itch their way down my cheek.

*You are invited
to a piano recital
May 25, 1985,
featuring the students
of Pamela Nielsen.*

*The performance will
take place in the
Beesley Music Center,
9400 South, 700 East,
Sandy, Utah,
at 10 a.m.*

*Please be prompt.*

My fingers were trembling as they dropped the quarter into the slot. It's ridiculous to be so shaky, I thought. They said it was simple. Just routine emergency gall bladder surgery.

She caught the phone on the first ring with a crisp, "Hello."

"Susan," I said, "This is Kathleen and I need to ask . . . "

"What's the matter?" she interrupted.

"Nothing, nothing. Everything's fine. It's just that I'm over at the hospital because Dave is going to have his gall bladder out, and I wanted to ask . . . "

Cutting in again, she demanded, "Are you alone?"

"Yes, but I'm okay. I just need to . . . "

Again insisting, "I'll be right there. Where are you?"

"No, no, that's not necessary."

"Listen, I'm coming over. I have some needlework to finish. I'll just sit."

"Okay," I gave in.

Hanging up the phone I wondered why I was feeling such relief to know someone was coming. Someone I didn't even know all that well. What was happening? Why was I on the verge of tears? I thought I had everything under control.

Dave had only come in for more ulcer tests because his abdomen had been giving him a little more pain this past week. Last night when I'd gone to pick him up after the tests and had found him registered in a room, I had been so surprised – and all he had done was complain about the anticipated loss of a week's work. Well, that would soon be over, and so would the physical stress that had been bothering him for the past six weeks. Thank heavens they'd finally figured out the problem.

So why was I so frightened? He had told me not even to come to the hospital. I had dismissed his request and had spent the previous evening soliciting friends to cover for me. Mike and Lynette would pick up all three children and take them to Kristen's piano recital. That would be going on right now. And then Linda was going to take Scott's fourteenth birthday group to the movie for me, and I would pick them up afterwards. It had been midnight when I'd tracked her down at a friend's house to set things up. No wonder I'm buzzed today.

But how had Dave changed so much overnight? When I'd walked into the room this morning his color had been so different I almost hadn't recognized him.

**Nielson, David R.**

**May 25, 1985**

It has been determined that there will be no surgery on Mr. Nielson until there is further evaluation. He is scheduled for a gastrointestinal workup to be conducted on May 26.

I slowly turned over and looked at the clock. Two a.m. In two more hours it would be six o'clock in Cleveland. That's still early for a holiday morning, but if George and Janice hadn't left town for the Memorial Day weekend that shouldn't be too obscene a time to call. Being a doctor, George would be used to it anyway.

I stared again at the ceiling, barely able to make out the swirls in the plaster's design. Somewhere in the house a light had been left on and my room was dimly illuminated with an eerie glow. My eyes caught the riveting stares from family pictures on one wall. They penetrated the night with questions. Having no answers I turned my back. My gaze fell on my open closet, and its disorganization shrieked at me; I turned again toward the ceiling.

I knew that sleep would never come and my mind kept opening little compartments of the past: the time in Seattle when Dave had been flying in Southeast Asia and the children and I had gone to my brother's for Christmas, the birth of our first child when friends had driven me to the hospital, and the only other sleepless night I'd ever had when, at twelve, I had broken my elbow.

Three a.m. I try to rehearse what I'm going to say to George. Nothing seems right. I am so tired I can barely raise my buzzing head. I need to make some decisions. I can't do it alone. Everyone has said they'll support what I decide. I don't want to decide. But no one will help me. I have to do something! George will help me know how to analyze it. He can tell me how to talk to the doctors. They're so impersonal. They talk around us. They aren't our friends. Why did our doctor have to be gone this weekend?

Dave is scared half to death by the surgeon on call. He even told me that if I decide to let him have surgery here he didn't want that guy to touch him! Well, that was one decision already made.

But what about the list of doctors his brother has given me? I don't want to call anyone. I want it all to go away. I want everyone to just go away. Dave can't be as sick as they say. He doesn't even feel bad.

People have been pouring into the hospital to see him. They must have announced it in church. We've felt like the main attraction at the circus. I guess I'm glad they came. I feel so alone now. I wish I could call them to come over.

Three-fifty a.m. That's close enough.

"George, it's Kathleen. I have something I need to talk to you about. It's going to be real hard to get it out, so please be patient."

"Is it the children? One of the kids?"

"No," I choked. "It's Dave."

"A car wreck! Has he been hurt bad?"

"No, no," I sobbed. "They tell me he's going to die. There is a large tumor on his pancreas."

The line was quiet. I had finally said it. Now it truly existed.

"Give me the details," he said.

I launched into an explanation of the events covering the last few days and finished by telling him that I just needed to know how to talk to the doctors.

"Hang on," he said, "I'll call you back in a couple of hours with some information." Leaning back on my pillow I could see the earliest light of day on the horizon. Already the eerie cast in my bedroom was gone.

A new day was coming, and a new phase of life was beginning.

May 25, 1985

*Dear Kathleen and Dave,*

*Just want you to know that we are thinking about you. We have not called or come to see you because we have been afraid of inconveniencing you. But if there is anything at all that we can do, please don't hesitate to call. We really want to help, and remember that we are never too busy.*

*Wish there were something we could do to ease your burden, and we hope and pray and know that everything will be fine for all of you in the long run, because you do have a Heavenly Father who loves you.*

Love,

Liv

Hospital *Pathology.* The sign on the door seemed harmless enough. And yet I knew that on the desk, in the file, or within the lab was the answer. The declaration of our future. The diagnosis. The announcement of what we would have to look forward to. Why were the doctors all so pessimistic? Even if the chances were a million to one against the tumor being benign, to me it was a fifty-fifty chance. It either was or it wasn't. So any chance at all meant that it could be okay and they'd operate and take it out.

Isn't that why we were going to Cleveland in the morning? So that the best hands in the business could do their duty? Until that very moment when the eyes of the surgeon were cast upon the mass no one would really know.

I opened the door and walked into the small outer office that housed the secretary, her desk, and a few chairs for waiting. It was near the end of the working day, and several people from inner offices were hurrying out with books and papers in hand. I sat down hoping for a moment's reprieve from the day's panic. I was there to pick up the pathology report of the breakdown of Dave's tumor cells. The hospital where the surgery was to be performed had requested that we bring all the information we could with us. My day's mission had been to gather X-rays, test results, and doctors' notes.

I took a deep breath and wished for another time, another circumstance. Take me back a week I thought, a month, or a year. Let me know what it's like to be free of this vise that is pressing on me from all sides. Let me breathe without quaking and relax without trembling.

What was happening to me? I couldn't even remember the last time I'd eaten, and that morning the bathroom scale had registered six fewer pounds. I probably had not slept more than eight hours adding all of the last five nights together.

I seemed to be functioning in a kind of daze. I felt like an observer most of the time, and I could see my parents at my home cooking, cleaning, caring for my children. And there I was, as if in slow motion, driving to the hospital, visiting Dave, talking to the doctors, driving back, making calls, checking on details.

And the phone, always ringing. I was so grateful for the concern, the empathy, the love, and yet saying the truth of what was happening over and over again made it seem even more unreal. Can that be me I hear saying those things? Cancer! What an ugly, threatening word.

I also wondered if that had been me I had seen a few hours before hollering at the clerk in the hospital where the original ultrasound films had been taken. She had been nice enough to explain that they were technically hospital property and, no, I could not have them, but they could be sent on to an address in Cleveland. I don't know what I said to her, but I probably would be embarrassed if I could remember. Her face was red when she stood up from her chair, and the woman who brought out the films and handed them to me was someone I hadn't seen before. As I had walked back to the car, I hated having made a scene. But at least I hadn't had to physically tear the place to pieces and the insisting *had* gotten results.

Breaking into my reverie, the pathologist came out of his office and motioned for me to join him within. He was very matter-of-fact with his information, and I thought that this was a real point-getter for the other team. My side was still in the huddle and the opponent was scoring wildly.

"The lab results were bad. The worst," he said, "It's the fastest growing kind of cancer cell. It will do crazy things. It will not be controlled. Has anyone really told you what's happening here?"

Here it comes again, I whispered to myself. The other team is scoring. Why do they have such an advantage? "You tell me," I said. "What's your opinion?"

"He's going to die, and soon. In the last five months I have diagnosed six pancreatic cancers. Five of them are now dead. Your husband is the sixth."

"Thank you," I mumbled, and got up to go. "We are going to Cleveland in the morning for surgery."

"Why?" he asked, surprised.

"Because he's forty-two years old," I blurted. "He's never been sick before, and we are able to afford it. We want to do everything within reason that we can. We have to be able to feel we gave it our best shot. And we know it's the only chance, however small it might be."

I braced myself for his next statement. He drew back and quietly said, "Well, good luck."

As I made my way to the car I had a feeling he was well aware of the score, and I began to wonder if I would know when to call "time out." Would there be a time when enough was enough and giving in would be preferable to a good showing?

The doctor who had done the endoscopy had already expressed his philosophy on the subject. Two days earlier he had sat me down in that cold, white room where he'd done the scope test and had extracted the piece of tissue they'd been analyzing.

"Listen," he had said. "If it were me. If it were my family, I'd want them to take me home and let me die. It wouldn't take long and I recommend no treatment. You have no idea how terrible this death will be."

At the time I had wanted to jump up and scream, how dare you inflict your judgments upon me! How dare you suggest that we give up! We can't just give in! We won't! I had said nothing.

So now I'd heard it again. It appears that our ballgame is fixed. Could it be I was just not listening to the coach's directions? What kind of a playoff were we headed for? Did we just not want to believe the facts?

ITINERARY

David and Kathleen Nielson

United Airlines Flight # 237

Date: 29 May 1985

LV: Salt Lake City 7:25 a.m.

AR: Cleveland 1:32 p.m.

*May 30, 1985*

*Dave,*

*My feelings of what a great guy you are were reinforced many times over when this bad luck hit. It seems like everyone had to comment on it. People feel like you have your act together and do things right.*
*I feel our relationship is comfortable, fun, and something I always learn from.*

*Thanks,*

*Jon R. Young*

*P.S. Lola, Kathleen's friend who's staying with the kids while you're in Cleveland, used to date my cousin Phil from Halfway, Oregon.*

I'm not going to lose control. I am going to keep my head about me. I am not going to let this take me down.

When Janice picks me up for lunch today I am going to have a good time. We will go to a nice, quiet restaurant. It will be decorated with soft, cool colors and the other patrons will be calmly conversing.

We will talk about bringing the children out to Cleveland. We will talk about how having us all together will be less stressful. Maybe we can even discuss taking the children to a park or the lake.

From the menu I will order a nutritious and delicious selection, maybe some seafood or a sandwich with cheeses and avocados. When the food comes I will eat it. It will taste good and it will give me energy. We will even order dessert. Chocolate! Something chocolate. That will be good. And I will feel okay that I am doing something ordinary. Having lunch with a friend.

Then after dessert we will talk about something in the future. Something I can look forward to. I have to somehow believe my life is not ending. It's not. It really isn't. It will go on, and there must be things to look forward to. Janice can tell me about some of those things. She can help me think of something ahead.

Cars! That's it. We will talk about cars. If or when I should buy a new car. Yes! That's it. I will think about getting a new car. We can look at the cars around us on the road. We can talk about the colors, the sizes, the different models.

I can see it now. A small van for traveling. The three children with me tripping from coast to coast, border to border . . . better yet, a sports car. There I go, hair flying, scarf trailing in the wind. Something small, fast, and red . . . or maybe a luxury car. I've always wanted a comfortable car with soft, deep seats, and an ultra-quiet ride . . . perhaps it should be a four-wheel drive so that we can go skiing anytime we want, and I wouldn't have to depend on the neighbors to help me get up our snowy hill in the winter.

What am I thinking about? This is almost exciting! I must be crazy! My husband is dying and I'm thinking about cars.

I know. After lunch we'll go shopping. I'll look for something to wear, or something to take home to the house as a memento of the trip.

Maybe we should just go for a ride and see some pleasant scenery. Yes, that would be good, just for a change of scene from the hospital.

Janice will be here soon, and we will go to a nice, cool place to eat, and then we will go for a pleasant ride before I go back to the hospital . . . maybe it wouldn't hurt to just look around and see what kinds of cars people are out and about in.

June 13, 1985

RE: Mr. David Nielson
CL: 1-785-755-1

Dear Dr. − − − :

I am writing in regard to Mr. David Nielson whom I have recently seen . . . for a rapidly developing abdominal and back pain, weight loss, and obstructive jaundice. A CT scan showed a mass in the pancreas.

I operated on Mr. Nielson on May 31, 1985. Unfortunately, I found a very large tumor mass at the head of the pancreas with. . . .

His eyes were opened wide as he threw me an agitated look. Nearly shouting, he said, "Are the children ready to go?"

Not knowing exactly what he meant, I mumbled an, "I guess so." I was hoping he wouldn't hear me and the conversation would be dropped.

"What do you mean?" he retorted. I could tell this was not going to end quickly. "Aren't their suitcases packed?" He was angry now, and his voice was taking on a surly tone.

"Yes," I answered calmly. "Their suitcases are packed." Praying that there would not be a confrontation, I held my breath in anticipation of what might come next.

"Then wake them up! Get them out of that bed!" I could see lines in his neck now where the muscles were tightening and the blood vessels in his temples were beginning to protrude. He seemed filled with anger, and the words came pouring out like water from an old-fashioned pump that has been primed and will empty all it has stored before it begins to subside. "Get the children downstairs! Can't you see we're going to be late? Do it now! Hurry!"

I blocked the rush of sounds by telling myself, "He doesn't know what he's saying. Just hang on. It will pass."

The room was silent until the next outburst. He looked up at the television high on the wall and said, "You'd better get the kids off TV or you'll never be ready to go."

Suddenly, the absurdity of the whole conversation came crashing down on me. I smiled in spite of his seriousness and said that it was okay. Everything was under control and he didn't have to worry. He closed his eyes and went to sleep.

I stood up from the chair beside his bed and walked to the hospital window to look out at the healthy world.

It was a beautiful, summer day, and in the outside world life didn't seem to be skipping a beat. I could see golfers on a nearby course wiping their sweaty brows, joggers running by on the street below, and a few players enjoying a game of tennis on some courts in the distance. They all seemed the picture of health.

I turned back toward his bed with thoughts of the doctor's words, "The delirium and disorientation are due to the hyper-calcium. The brain is becoming calcified, but if the count comes down the disorientation will disappear." I wondered how long it would last, and when the prognosis was fulfilled – "Death due to terminal cancer" – would it bring welcome relief or just more pain?

June 14, 1985

Dear Mother and Dad,

I know you've been really concerned about the financial implications of Dave's illness. Now that we're back from Cleveland I've been able to sort it out a little and it looks okay right now.

Dave made enough money this spring to keep us the rest of the year if we are careful. The insurance will be covering close to 100% of the doctor and hospital bills now that the deductible is paid, so we're fine there.

When I cleaned off my desk yesterday I found the application for disability insurance. How I wish we'd sent it in. If you're self-employed it's really stupid to not have it. Hindsight, I guess.

Well, I wish I could say we are all fine. We are all adjusting. It's just such a nightmare. Love you and miss you. Thanks for all the help and support when you come here.

Love,

Kathleen

Decisions, decisions. Every time I turn around there are more decisions. Surgery. Do we have it, or do we go home and wait? Then, who will do it and where? Who will look after the children? How much treatment should be allowed? Should we attempt relief through the pain clinic again? And now this one.

They came into the hospital room and spoke with me when Dave was out being X-rayed. Like a division of recruits the five of them in white stood at the foot of his bed staring at me, waiting for an answer. I remained glued to my chair by the window, wanting to look outside or go back to my magazine. Maybe they'll just fade away, I thought. I don't want to do this today.

They kept pushing as though there was some urgency about the decision. The chief resident was doing most of the talking, but his entourage of interns continued to nod in agreement. Was it really that significant?

He was dying anyway. We all knew that. Then I listened more carefully and began to comprehend its importance. "You see, it isn't pleasant what we would have to do. You have to understand the procedure that we go through in the event there's a cardiac arrest."

A picture began to form in my mind. I could see Dave's poor, sick body being pounded on, jerked around, and . . . and . . . I knew they were correct. I think it is sometimes referred to as "the right to die."

It seemed strange to me that they would even think of reviving him under the circumstances. I guess it's policy or law or something that they would have to revive a patient in an emergency. If I were not there or had not officially requested that no reviving be done, they were saying, they'd have to do everything they could to sustain his life. Then the question of maintaining life support would come into play. The clearing picture made my decision obvious.

"There are papers you'll have to sign," they were saying.

"Okay, okay, tomorrow."

As they left I wondered why this decision seemed so hard. It shouldn't be. His fate was already determined. Is it just that I didn't want to have the final say?

Department of Nutritional Services

Name: *David R. Nielson*

Clinic Number: *1-785-755-1*

Date: *6/15/85*

Diet: *Nutritional Guidelines for
    Cancer Patients*

My life has stopped. It is suspended, dangling from a fraying string that is stretched between the past and the future. It hangs constant in time, neither progressing nor regressing, and watches the lives of others go marching by.

My life has taken on the sole role of caretaker, and like a faithful sentinel that has forsaken any personal pursuits, has committed itself to only the one cause. As my life performs the duties relevant to the assignment, it turns away from any compulsion toward other desires that loom up from within. Doused are the fires of life, the freedoms that we enjoy, the simple things we take for granted. Buried are the urges to dance, to sing, and to love. These basics have been replaced by fear, worry, and despair.

My life stands on guard and knows not what it is waiting for. Goals are undefined and the job description changes daily. Happenings in the rest of the world are heralded through the media to fall upon my deaf ears, muted by my single-minded-ness. My life hears only one song and the melody is chaotic. The music is constantly changing pace. It searches desperately for a direction, a command, and begs for relief.

The fraying string supporting my lifeline tightens and relaxes with the changes in the weather. Sometimes the wind brings stresses that stretch the line to breakpoint. Other times the stillness that surrounds my life in the absence of turbulence can only resemble the calm before the storm, and my life stands poised to accept the impending doom.

While this state of limbo exists, time for others has moved along. Vacations have been taken. Employments have changed. Houses have been built. Babies have been born.

How do the passersby view my position? Do they know with what deep heartfelt desires my life longs for the familiarity of their mundane schedules? Do they comprehend the anger and frustration that ensues from my not marching alongside them? Is the mask my life has constructed sufficiently hiding the pain?

But a bigger storm is coming. My life will continue only after it blows over. The fraying string holding my life in suspension will tighten and flex and the activity will be unnoticed by the passing crowd. How far will they travel? Will my life be out of step when it seeks to join the throng, or will it be picked up and carried along?

Insurance Administrators

Employee Benefit Specialists

Prescription Drug Program

0597  1514  52976543

043 PCS

D R Nielson

06/19/85            C18            3.00

"What happened last night? The room is a mess!" I was standing beside Dave's hospital bed. He turned toward me with that "Who in the hell are you?" look in his eyes.

There was blood all over the I.V. stand. Then I saw it on the floor. It wasn't just a little bit. Every couple of steps there were reddish-black spots, and in between there were little drops of the same color. It had probably happened sometime in the night because the fluid had already been totally absorbed into the hard-finish gray carpet. I thought that maybe I'd stepped on some of it when I'd come in and I wanted to clean off the bottoms of my shoes. I was looking for a tissue when I noticed that Dave had dried blood on his hands and arms. It was stiff on his skin and was creasing and flaking off his knuckles. I only then realized that the blood on the floor must be his. I hurried into the small bathroom to get a wet washcloth, and when I switched on the light I had to grab the door frame to steady myself. As though it had been spilled from a container held high, blood splashes were everywhere. The floor of the small shower stall had collected much of it, and the curtain itself had long drying drips of the telltale dark red.

I stayed in the small cubicle long enough to convince the roll in my stomach to subside, dampened a washcloth, and returned to Dave's bed to wipe his hands clean.

I knew that questioning him would go nowhere. I wasn't sure he even knew who I was, let alone what had happened during the night. Instead, I hurried to the nurses' station.

The terse excuses I got were little consolation for the wife of a dying man. "Housekeeping will get to it. We were short-handed last night." The staff's inability to answer the more important question of what had actually happened was even more distressing. No one could pin down the activity exactly, but apparently sometime in the early morning hours he had gotton out of bed and had wandered into the bathroom. As he had moved away from the bed he had pulled out his catheter and I.V.s and had begun to bleed.

I hated them all. I didn't care for one second that they were over-worked and under-staffed. It was my husband's life we were dealing with, and I was fast losing my ability to cope. I forced myself to push down the anger and frustration and stayed in control only because I knew that I would be seeing a lot of this hospital staff during the next few weeks. We compromised and they quickly brought in a new I.V. stand, promising that someone would come to clean the bathroom. They did, but it took five days before they got to the spots on the floor, and I was reminded of the episode whenever I looked down.

Dave, meanwhile, seemed oblivious to the whole experience. His I.V. and catheter had been replaced, and he had received a blood transfusion to replace the lost blood. They put up the rails on the sides of his bed.

The doctors were now concerned that he would hurt himself again. To the disgruntlement of the night nursing staff, a friend or relative was to stay with him at night until he was once again rational and coherent.

During my time on guard I wondered how much physical suffering he had actually endured. When the mind is altered as his had been by the calcium, how much does one really experience? Was it painful when he had ripped the tubes out? Did he cry out unheard? Was he trying to leave and come home? The questions would never be answered. Just knowing that he couldn't remember would have to be comfort enough.

**Nielson, David R.**   #55-65-01/5

Date

7/19/85   Mr. Nielson returns today for day 28 chemotherapy in his FAM program. In the interim he required a three-day hospitalization because of nausea, vomiting, and beginning dehydration. With modification of his anti-nausea medication to include Reglan, this had cleared, and he appears to be eating better. He has gained four pounds since his last visit here and reports no further vomiting, although he continues to have difficulty with his appetite.
His pain control is reasonably good. He has no worsening.
**PHYSICAL EXAMINATION:** He is a chronically ill man who is beginning to lose his hair. He is not jaundiced. The lungs are clear. The vital signs are normal. The abdominal exam continues to show the massive tumor area, which, as near as I can tell, is unchanged. . . .

The neighbor was just checking when she came over. Checking with the usual, "How are you? Is there anything I can do to help?" The questions that are so often stated and sometimes meant.

We were standing on the front porch, and as she was rattling on with the nervous prattle of one who thinks a silent moment should be filled with sound, I smiled and nodded, physically looking at her and at the same time looking past her. I noticed the grass needed to be cut, weeds were invading the marigolds, and there were some pieces of a paper plate caught in the pyracantha.

How long had it been since we had seeded the grass, bought the shrubs, and planted the trees? We had always done everything together. Memories! Memories! Would I always be plagued with pictures of him in my mind, bending over the dirt as he made sure the seed was being evenly distributed, pushing and pulling on the rocks to make sure their placement was just right, standing with hands on hips bitching at me when I wanted the last tree moved twelve inches to the right?

Suddenly I was jerked back to the neighbor's conversation. What was that? What had she said? My mind raced to clarify her statement. I repeated it to myself wondering what could possibly have prompted such a question. "Don't you sometimes just wish it were all over with?"

How could I want it to be over with? And yet, there was a ring of truth in what she had said. I did want to be relieved of the constant vigil, watching him deteriorate day by day. I did so desperately want to be back in my old role of mother, helpmate, and lover. But how could that be?

If he died and it were all over with, as she had put it, I couldn't be the mother I'd been because I'd have to be the father, too. I couldn't be a helpmate because there would be no mate, and my bed would be empty.

These changes even now seemed the hardest. I was already playing both roles. And even though the bed wasn't empty, it was barely warm and thoughts of lovemaking had long since been put aside. How different could it be?

But it's the sense of belonging, isn't it? We belonged to each other. We were there for each other. The role was defined. I knew how to make him happy. I knew how to love him. We were used to each other. We'd grown up together. Now that was all changing, and I didn't like the change. But I knew what was expected. There was a certain comfort in that. And while I didn't know how long we could endure the present situation, the thought of being alone, being without a husband's love, and being a single parent in a neighborhood of families was noxious to me.

Thinking of her question again, I smiled at my well-meaning neighbor. Pushing back the reality that it would be over whether I wished for it or not, I said, "Well, sometimes I think about what it would be like."

July 30, 1985

Dear Kathleen,

I was sitting around feeling kind of blue, wishing you were closer so we could sit around and have a Coke and talk! I hate living in such a rush that I don't have time for old friends.

Anyway, I miss you and love you all. I'm just so glad that I was able to come down and stay with the kids while you and Dave were in Cleveland.

XOX to Dave

XOX to that cute and funny Kristen

XOX to Scott, my sweetie and a big OXO to Ryan.

And to you, my dear friend, my same ole true blue friendship.

Love,

Lola

Why can't I hold still? I keep moving, pacing, running from one room to another. Why can't I concentrate on one task at a time? I just put a load of laundry in the washer. Was that hours ago? I remember taking the vacuum upstairs. I think it was yesterday. And the dishes. I can't seem to get anything done.

What am I waiting for? Is the phone going to ring and the doctor say, "It's all a mistake!" No. Is the body lying in my bed going to emerge whole and well after its rest? No. Are the hospital bills going to stop filling my mailbox? No.

Where will it end? We are sinking. Sinking. As Dave's life is slowly ebbing away, mine is being sucked out of me by a giant octopus. Its tentacles have encircled my body, twisting and pulling at my every move. I can't seem to get out of its grip. I wake in the morning smothered by its mass, and as my day goes on, I struggle beneath its crushing strength. I rush from task to task, dragging it from room to room, desperately trying one thing after another to loosen its hold on me.

Am I wishing Dave's condition were worse? Maybe if he had one more setback he could go to the hospital, and then I could stop running. I would sleep for twenty-four hours or go to bed with a book. I could leave him there for at least one day without me. But then I would go, and the children would be alone again. The tentacles would tighten and the frustration level would rise. I would need to be in both places. No. It's better that he's home.

But I can't stand it! There's no relief! Inside I'm screaming, "It's not fair! Not to him. Not to the children. Not to me." I know, I know, no one said it would be fair. But is there ever a balance?

Will the day come when my octopus withdraws? Will its tentacles ever loosen and slip away? And if they do, how bruised will I be? What scars will remain? How long will it take me to be whole again?

August 12, 1985

Re: David R. Nielson

Dear Dr. – – – ,

Your patient David Nielson was again admitted to the Medical Center on August 5th and was discharged on the 9th. He again was admitted because of intractable nausea. . . . You will recall that he had an episode of this just several weeks ago.

He was discharged on August 9th at his request to attend a family wedding and reunion, and, hopefully, to return to eating small meals at regular intervals. He was given a followup appointment. . . .

We will keep you informed of his progress, but his prognosis is obviously guarded.

Thank you for sending him here.

I didn't recognize the woman's voice, and when she asked to speak to Kristen, I was curious. Informing her that Kristen was not home, I asked if I could take a message. She answered, "No," and seemed anxious to end the conversation.

"Who might I say is calling?" I inquired.

Hesitantly she replied that she was with Hospice of Salt Lake.

"Oh!" I said, feeling a little relieved. "It's not Kristen you want, it's me, Kathleen. I'm the wife of the patient."

"Yes, I know," she replied and went on somewhat reluctantly. "I'm calling to speak with Kristen."

Immediately my concern level began to rise, and I asked her why she would be calling my sixteen-year-old daughter.

"Actually," she hesitated, "I'm returning her call from yesterday."

An alarm was going off in my head, yet still disbelieving I said, "There must be some mistake. Why would Kristen call you?"

"She called in tears," the woman responded. "She said she didn't know what to do, that she had to talk with someone and she had called us because she knew we had met with you."

I have let her down, I thought. I have only been concerned with Dave and myself, and making sure Ryan is cared for. Kristen and Scott, teenagers, need more attention. What was I going to do? How could I help them?

"What did she say?" I pleaded.

"She said she couldn't approach you because you had so much to deal with already, but that she was so upset it frightened her."

I was stunned. This had been going on and I hadn't even seen it. Was I now so narrowly tuned that I was missing something this important? Or was Kristen just a master at disguising her emotions?

"Were you able to help her?" I queried.

"I was on the phone with her for some time yesterday, and she seemed to settle down and be okay. I told her I would check into counseling possibilities at the high school, and I'm calling back with the information now."

"Thank you," I said. "Perhaps you could call back in an hour and speak with her. I rather think she would not like me to know or she would have told me herself. I appreciate your help and follow-through." I hung the phone back on its wall perch and sank onto the bench beside it.

The phone's long dangling cord was gently swinging in a small arc back and forth along the wall. The cord, like my life, had been stretched and twisted and knotted. Some of the curlicues in the cord were backwards and others were bunched together creating a pattern of weird shapes. In between, stretches of the cord hung loose, barely resembling the original tight-ringed, precise design it had once displayed.

I remembered how Dave used to stand on a chair sometimes and dangle the phone down from an outstretched hand to get the tangles out. The phone would spin and spin, unraveling the maze of curlicues. How I wish someone could simply spin me through my paces to emerge in a straightened-out form, myself.

Getting up, I noticed a blue and white pamphlet tacked on the bulletin board above the bench. "Hospice of Salt Lake," with the phone number in bold print. I was proud that she had had the good sense to turn to someone capable of giving real help.

We had only had two Hospice visits, and I couldn't even remember if Kristen had met the nurse who had come out. Shortly after Dave's diagnosis I had been briefed by a friend about Hospice's role in the community, how it could offer relief to the family of the patient, and how through it's program it would be possible to keep someone at home who might otherwise need to be hospitalized.

When I had questioned the doctor about it he had quickly come back with, "Why would you want Hospice? It just helps out when the person is actually dying, right at the end." Puzzled, I looked

at him wondering what he thought was going on.
Either he didn't understand it's role as it had been
explained to me, or maybe he didn't actually
understand what it was like for a patient and his
family at home when death comes slowly. Those of
us who hovered about Dave, not knowing much of
the time what was happening medically, needed
accessible support.

So I had called Hospice and there had found a
friend – and attainable information I could
depend on. The problem was that Dave had balked
at the idea of strangers and had insisted that I be
the only one who attended to him. So for us
Hospice had remained simply the friend to call,
and only on rare occasions had been able to offer
palliative care.

It was a comfort to know that out of the snarl
of our lives Kristen had seen clearly enough to seek
counsel for herself.

# A BIRTHDAY PARTY

## #4

FOR:   *Ryan Nielson*

PLACE:  *Ryan's house*

DATE:   *August 19, 1985*

TIME:   *2 pm*

The photos were back from the developer and I tore open the package with the zeal of one who thinks he just might have taken the prize-winning shot. They were the prints of Ryan's fourth birthday party with five of his neighborhood friends as they had scrambled for their places in relay games and then had spread cake crumbs from one end of the kitchen to the other.

The picture of them all seated around the table caught my attention. It was the typical gathering. They were all seated half on their chairs, and each had one leg dangling downward reaching for the floor's security. Two of the girls were laughing while pointing fingers at the boy across from them whose face was arranged in a Draculan configuration, and one arm with spoon in hand was stretched across the table toward another's plate. I was smiling at the memory when the background reached out to me. The family room beyond the kitchen area was out of focus, but seated on the couch was the birthday boy's father. I had been so careful to avoid taking pictures of him. Someone had mentioned early on that we should do some video taping, but none of us had wanted that. For us it had been the right choice. From the moment of diagnosis he had become a stranger emotionally, and his body had quickly followed suit, changing in appearance until we had to remind ourselves that this was the daddy and the Dave we knew and loved.

But the birthday photograph burned a picture in my brain that refuses to leave. I set it aside after thinking about it and later tore it to shreds and destroyed the negative as well. And yet I still see him sitting there, clearer than the picture itself. The light-blue tee shirt with the mountain scene on the front was clinging to his body, and at the same time hanging. It clearly outlined the bony shoulder blades, the hunching back. His long, thin arms dangled from their attachment to the body as though without their proper connection. The elbows were bent with hands clasped across his lap, resting on his thighs. His hands seemed not still, as perhaps his fingers were moving, gently stroking one another, frustrated as they lay incapable of their tasks. His body suggested a gentle sway of movement, as if he did not quite have his balance. His head was bent, chin near chest, and gently nodded as the lids over his eyes had slipped to half mast. Dave's head, hairless now, had caught a little of the camera's flash, which further intensified the drastic physical changes.

I wondered if he had even been aware of the frolicking children, or if he had merely pooled all his strength into not letting their piercing voices and shouts penetrate his shroud. Whatever the case, he had tolerated it well, and feeling that he should make a showing, had done so.

# STAFF NOTES

David Nielson
55-65-01/5

7/26/85  Wt. 140# 63.5 kg
no dictation

8/20/85  Wt. 134# 60.8 kg

8/20/85  David has felt significantly improved. He is eating better, with a significantly increased overall food intake, but has not gained weight. . . . He reports no significant pain.

**PHYSICAL EXAMINATION**: He is a chronically ill-appearing, thin young man weighing 134 pounds. This represents a 26-pound weight loss since mid-June. . . .

**PLAN**: In view of his slow recovery from his previous GI distress . . . , we will hold his chemotherapy one additional week, at which time he will make an intensive trial of using the Viokase to see if he can begin to regain some weight and strength. He will return at that time for his second eight-week cycle of FAM chemotherapy since he has had more than a 50% reduction in the size of his tumor mass.

Dave slipped today as he was painstakingly mounting the stairs, and in the half second it took him to grasp with a firm enough hold to stabilize, I envisioned myself catching him and both of us tumbling head-over-heels to the bottom. The thought sent one of those chills through me that made my whole body jerk with a spasm. I found myself almost convulsing as I tried to shake away the mental picture. Pushing hard to remove the scene, my mind quickly responded to the rescue with the mind game it so often played now. The contest was to replace the picture of the revolting or agonizing situation at hand with a vision of the past and happier moments.

The memory I envisioned this time produced a chuckle that I smothered into a smile as I saw a healthy Dave ascending the stairs ahead of me. He instinctively reached behind him with both hands to cover and protect his vulnerable backside as my hand was closing in for the pinch. He jumped even before I made contact and practically hopped over the last three steps. It had been such a game with us, and over the years his defensive instincts had become very keen as my offensive maneuvers had become more ingenious and were often supported with surprise attacks.

Slipping back to the present, I looked above me at the baggy sweat pants that hung on the mere post of a man. The firm, tight cheeks were gone, and I thought of how quickly the body's tone and muscle structure dissipate and dissolve with illness and loss of weight. What a sadness the sight of his body invoked. Sometimes I even wondered who the stranger was. Did I know him? Other times I just wanted to put my arms around him and hold him like a child, rocking and swaying him to offer comfort. This was impossible, of course, because his physical pain prohibited any kind of hugging or squeezing and allowed only the slightest touching. And now as I thought again of having to catch him if he stumbled or fell, my thoughts were of how little protection he had covering his bones.

He seemed so fragile and brittle that we thought perhaps the slightest bumps would do immense damage. The children were all fearful that he would "turf it" just walking across the kitchen floor and break into a million pieces. The bones seemed to be sharp as well as brittle, and he often spoke of how he was constantly poked by his own structure.

Last week he had felt good enough to attend a movie, so we had all decided to go. I was elected to carry the pillows for him to sit on, and off we had gone. He had held up pretty well, but we knew he had never felt very comfortable and he had said afterwards that we should only see videos from now on.

Sitting had become very uncomfortable, as what weight he did have pressed his hip bones down on his thin rump so hard that he thought they'd go right through the skin. We had continued to carry a pillow with us wherever we ventured, but we stayed away from any sustained sitting.

My thoughts suddenly jumped back to the present, and I found he had reached the top of the stairs ahead of me. Momentarily losing his balance, he was flailing his arms in backward circular motions to regain the posture needed to proceed. I hung in the background not quite knowing when to offer physical assistance, but hoping to be close enough if it were needed. He gained control and headed for his destination, the couch by the television. It looked inviting with its soft, white cover, offering comfort even before he reached it. As he carefully lowered himself into a restful position I thought of how sure he was that things were getting better – how he assessed his strength every day, and, fearful that he would be incapacitated, felt that he was holding his own.

It frightened him sometimes when standing naked he would look into the mirror before getting into the shower. "I look like a Biafran refugee!" he'd say, and sure enough he did. But he continued to observe and analyze the progress optimistically. The desperate fight to gain weight just never seemed to be won. His shoulders and arms resembled those of an unclothed marionette, and his legs were mere sticks supporting a distended abdomen. "I'm doing okay, though," he'd summarize. "I just have to gain some weight."

Before I left him on the couch to watch the news, I realized again that it's not only the physical body that deteriorates with illness, but one's reasoning capabilities as well. Going back downstairs I played the mental game again and reflected upon his accomplishments of the past. So many times he had demonstrated the ability to realistically project where his work was going and how to guide his time and energy to a fruitful reward.

Thank heavens there were good times, I thought. I'm going to be pulling them out to examine for a long time to come.

*Dear Dave,*

*The other day at Mom and Dad's I noticed the picture she says is one of her favorites. You're holding the backstay of the 20 foot sailboat we rented in Tibron, and are wearing my black and brown Pendleton. I've got on a watch cap and am pointing to something with my crooked index finger. . . . Kathleen must have taken the picture with our Instamatic.*

*In the photo the sun is quite bright and there don't appear to be any clouds. Once away from the dock, though, we had white caps and a hard time staying clear of other boats. . . . There were boats everywhere and Kathleen was sure she'd never again see the baby daughter she'd left behind with a sitter at the Presidio VOQ where you were staying. . . .*

*I don't know if we ever got out as far as the bridge that day, but tacking back near Alcatraz we passed a flotilla of class boats flying spinnakers on a downwind course. You remarked that the wind was blowing the same way for all of us, but we were moving*

steadily in a variety of directions —
an echo of somebody's poem, "It's not
the gales, but the set of the sails. . . . "
    You were training in jets then,
two years married to my little sister,
and I was in my first year of law
school. When we got back to Tibron
everyone had on somebody else's
jacket.

Love,

David

I can't seem to sleep much. At night I lie with my cheek pressed against the cool sheet, and staring into the darkness wonder if my eyes are open or closed. Blinking, I realize they're open, but there seems to be no difference. The nightmare continues whether I escape through slumber or not.

I can hear his breathing breaking the quiet of the night. It is slightly labored and uneasy. Though not loud, its irregular pattern shatters the stillness. I put a pillow over my head and hope the hum of the silence I feel from its pressure will drown out the rasp of his light puffing. When I can hear the pounding of my heart I withdraw the covering and try to relax.

I long for the nights when we slept clasped in each other's arms and to be awakened in the early morning darkness by the other's desires was a sweet interruption of a full night's sleep.

Believing that part of our life is over, my mind springs to those memories to push away the present. Longing for that closeness of another time, I stretch out my arm toward him and carefully slip it under his pillow. There I can feel the weight of his presence and know that he is close. To actually touch him would only destroy the moment and he too would wake into the night's frightful reality.

My fingers stroking and tracing patterns on his skin only bring discomfort to him now. Their caress is no longer welcome. It is as though his whole being meditates, trying mentally to drive away the evils invading his body. My touch is a distraction, an intrusion from another life that calls for a response that is now foreign to him.

Regretfully understanding his lack of desire for intimacy, I settle for memories of the past and think of how life used to be, the awkwardness of newlyweds, the gratifying weekend get-aways from children, and the relaxing ease of a long-lasting, mature relationship.

His breathing quickens and I withdraw my hand. I raise myself on my elbow poised to rush and assist. I am fearful that his nausea has returned or that the pain has worn through the medication and his discomfort will require more attention. However, he is merely restless and soon struggles into a position that gives him comfort. The short, raspy breaths are once again the only sounds as the rustling bedclothes settle gently around him.

Looking in his direction I can still see only darkness, but envision the person beside me. He has changed physically so much that I wonder what I'd do if he actually did make a sexual advance. I find myself repulsed at the very thought and a quiver travels the length of my body.

I recall the doctor's consoling words. "You'll just have to be patient and understanding. As he gets healthier and stronger the desires will return."

We were standing in the hallway of the cancer clinic while Dave was getting a treatment in the next room. At the time I had thought that my sexual desires had fled as well, and I had merely asked if it were possible that Dave might want to have sex in the condition he was in. The first remarks from the doctor had shocked me, as he had quickly looked up, making sure I fully understood his intent, and had cautioned, "There cannot be a pregnancy. You must use protection in any case. A pregnancy would be a disaster. It would almost surely be aborted due to the chemotherapy and must be avoided. The probability of conception is extremely low, but the risk is too great to disregard the possibility." By the time he had gotten to the part about my being understanding, I was hoping the opportunity would never come to me.

I wondered why we used poisons to sustain life that in turn would destroy it. I questioned the validity of tampering with something that could alter the body's reproductive system, the very essence of being. The puzzle was getting more complex as I tried to interpret each piece of information that came my way. These thoughts of sex had provoked a whole new area, and I was unsure how to handle the information.

Lying in bed now beside Dave, I try to think of his needs and wonder how I could ever deny an advance from him. And yet I know within me I do not want to carry that memory. I feel selfish harboring these thoughts, but I can only imagine that the comparison with our healthy life would simply bring one more heartache.

Trying to relax, I wonder if the doctor's comment, "As he gets healthier and stronger the desires will return," could mean that when he's healthier and stronger my desires will return as well. I guess it's just one more piece that doesn't fit yet. There's no way of knowing right now how either of us would react. I hope we'll both be patient and understanding.

*September 15, 1985*

*Dear Dave and Kathleen,*
  *We wanted you both to know that our thoughts and prayers are with you. We feel horrified, shocked, and angry that such an unfair thing is happening to people who we care about as friends. As you both continue to deal with this, we pray that you will both find the inner strength, the peace and the comfort to guide you through this difficult period.*

  *Love,*
  *Chris and Lee*

"**I** have to see the children before we leave," he pleaded, and I turned to see fear in his expression.

"What's wrong?" I asked.

"I just have to see them before we go to the hospital."

"Dave, you're okay," I reassured him. "You need to be hydrated because you are so sick right now, but this will pass. I'll go get the children if you want, but they aren't home. They've gone with the neighbors somewhere. I promise, you'll be okay this time. It isn't over yet. This is not the end." I couldn't believe what I was saying. It had just come out.

"Well, let's just go then."

The emergency room had been warned about our coming, but a major accident had set them back. They put us in a small room where the air-conditioner was set in the arctic zone, and I quickly became more concerned about Dave's condition. He seemed tense and uneasy. An I.V. team had been ordered to get him set up, but they hadn't arrived yet. I wrapped him in blankets I found in a cupboard in the hallway, but he kept shivering.

I stood beside the gurney he lay on and bent over him, carefully encircling his upper body with my arms. Quietly he began to sob. "I'm so afraid," he murmured. I had never known him to cry. Not once in the eighteen years we'd been together. I didn't know what to say. I just stood there gently patting him.

"I'm afraid it will hurt," he said. "I just don't want it to be painful." Then tears came in shudders and I saw before me a little boy. A sad, frightened, little boy, who had done the best he could. One who had fought bravely and had still been beaten by the bully, the neighborhood kid who went around striking out indiscriminately at whomever he pleased. And the little boy standing by himself, bruised and swollen from the tussle, was looking at me with a tear-stained, dirty face. He didn't understand why.

"It hurts so bad," he was saying. "I just don't want it to hurt more."

I pulled away from him, wiping my own tears, and with an all-knowing emphasis pronounced, "It won't hurt, Dave. I don't know much about this, but I do know that death itself will not hurt."

**10/7/85**

We have prescribed oral morphine for Mr. Nielson, elixir of morphine 10 mg/ml, 30-40 mg. every 3-4 hours. This should give him complete relief.

I slowly pushed his wheelchair down the corridor. Questioning stares shot at us from those we passed. Onlookers smiled and nodded, possibly on missions of mercy themselves, but many sought after us with a more curious expression and sighed with relief as we passed. Those who gawked without reservation merely demonstrated the shock we all felt.

If only they could have known the whole man, I thought. This pathetic resemblance of him was such a contrast to the man I had lived and worked with. What a travesty our life had become, from one of excitement and energy to one of somber inactivity.

I stopped the wheelchair just short of the elevator's metal doors and stepped on the brake. Striving to hold on to what independence he could, Dave purposefully reached out his hand and pressed the "down" button. But rather than the frail, thin hands of a dying man, I saw the ones I had fallen in love with.

Suddenly I was back in college seated on the bleachers beside him as he took my hand in both of his. It was the first time he had touched me, and I had known immediately I liked him. His touch had been soft and gentle, yet firm and strong. I had envisioned him a leader, as his hold on me had told of commitment and purpose. I had felt I was in capable company. The softness had spoken of tender care, while the strength had suggested hard work. I had wanted to hold on tight.

One year later I had held the same hands, the hands of a jet pilot. "Golden," the jargon goes. He who has golden hands flies at the head of his class feeling the very essence of the aircraft, knowing instinctively how to handle a high-performance jet. Golden hands are always in control and at the same time reaching for the edge, the very peak of excellence.

Some years later I had handed nails to the hands of a carpenter. The same gentle, strong, golden hands. These hands had skillfully worked through heat and cold to build our home. Bruised and callused, they had continued to toil. Not so soft then, but still gentle with their touch. Firmer and stronger, they had worked to complete the task, the dream.

As life had matured, the hands had settled into the work they loved best. They had spent countless hours designing and building computer systems. The minute pieces and the intricate details had been conscientiously handled. And as some do, these hands had seen the fruits of their labors grow. They had seen projects completed and plans go into production.

In many ways these hands had been the hands of a lucky man. A man who had high goals and had been privileged to achieve them. Combined with his knowledge and energy, his hands had performed well for him. These hands, thin, frail, and lifeless now, bore little resemblance to the hands I had fallen in love with.

October 18, 1985

Mr. David Nielson

Dear Dave,
This letter will serve as written confirmation that we are unable to continue coverage for you under our medical plan. The 60-day sick leave that you had with . . . expired on October 1, 1985, and you have 30 days from that date to convert your policy with. . . .
Should you have any questions concerning this, please call me. . . .

Sincerely,

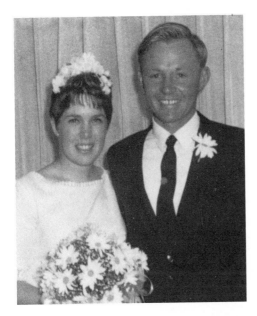

*Wedding, June 27, 1968.*

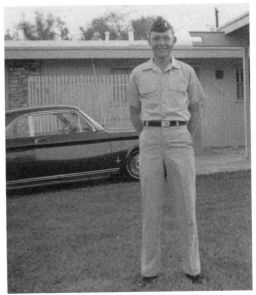

*A happy 2nd Lieutenant.*

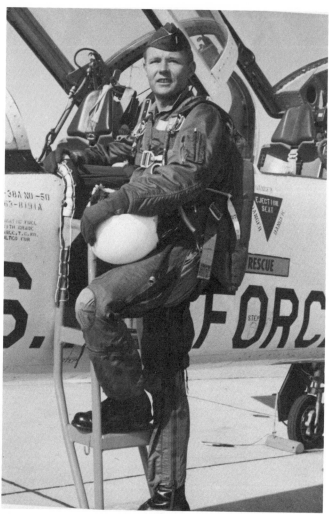

*Flight training, Williams AFB, AZ, 1969.*

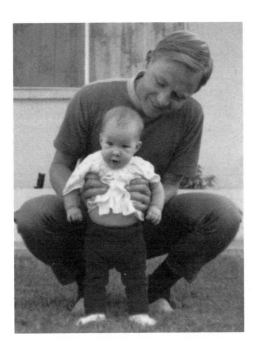

*Dave with baby Kristen, Chandler, AZ, 1969.*

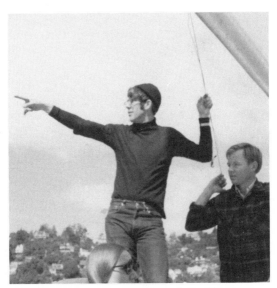

*Sailing on San Francisco Bay with Kathleen's brother, David, Spring 1970.*

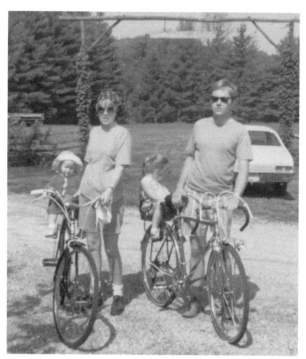

*Knawbone Camp, Brown County, IN, 1972.*

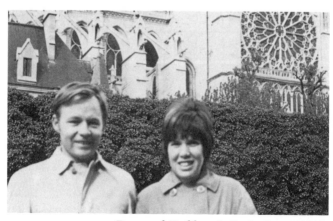

*Dave and Kathleen in Paris, Spring 1973.*

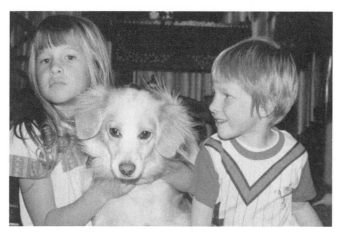

*Kristen and Scott with new pup, Duke, Sandy, UT, 1975.*

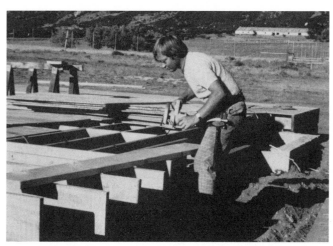

*House building, Summer 1978.*

*Halloween,
1979.*

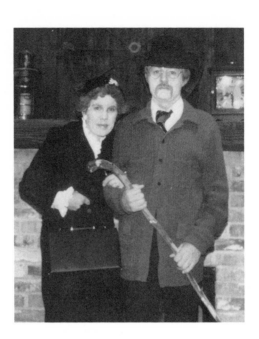

*McCall, ID, 1980, The smile we remember best.*

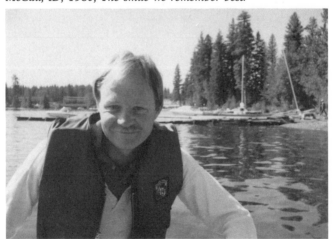

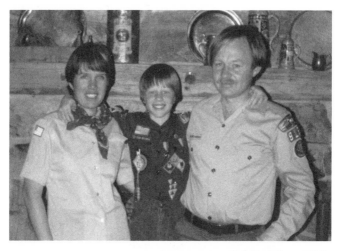

*Cub Scouting, 1981.*

*Under Niagara Falls, part of the 6,000 mile trip,
October 1982.*

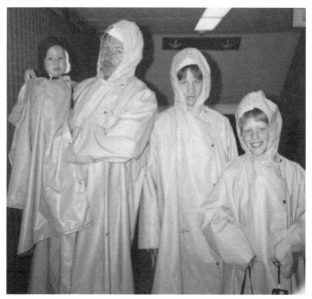

*Long Beach Harbor on the last family vacation,*
*November 1984.*

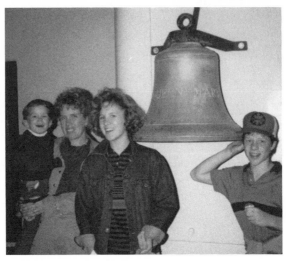

*Scott and Dave winning foot races at a father and son's*
*outing, May 18, 1985, seven days before diagnosis.*

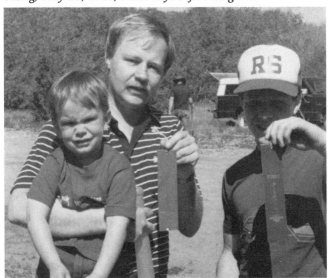

*Ryan's fourth birthday party, August 1985.*

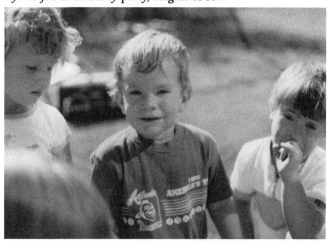

*Dave with Scott near St. George, UT, October 1985.*

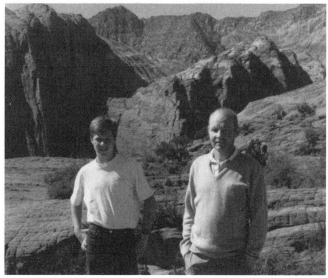

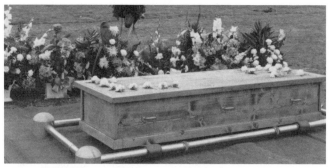

*January 22, 1986.*

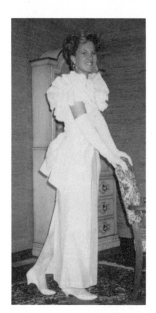

*Kristen going to the prom,
April 1986.*

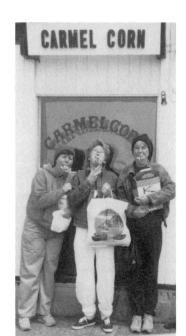

*Friend Lola, Kristen, and
Kathleen coming back to life
on the Oregon coast,
August 1986.*

The road stretched ahead of us like a dark gray ribbon threading itself through the sagebrush, among the scrubby juniper, and over the rocky terrain, rising and falling with the valleys and hills. The winter landscape offered little variety of color, and the blending of the grays and browns and darker grays and browns seemed to suggest the darkness in our lives.

It was the Thanksgiving school vacation, and we were returning home after a three-day visit with the grandparents. Once home we would renew our efforts and ride out the storm.

The tempest had raged wildly over the past weeks as Dave's illness had begun its final assault. The cancer had fought a true battle in every sense, charging ahead, then falling back in retreat only to hide and spring again from a new position, striking in a more vulnerable spot each time. Every attack had weakened the main party, and now as a fallen army straggles home to survey its losses, we were headed back to gear up for our final retreat.

We had left Dave at his brother's on Thanksgiving afternoon and had left for the grandparent's the following morning. The vacation had been a necessary diversion. I was wearing down, and the possibility of uninterrupted rest looked as good as a mirage in the desert. Fortunately, the diversion had fulfilled its promise, and I felt more capable of coping with the horror invading our lives.

As I drove along I became mesmerized by the drone of the car's engine, and the treeless landscape at times seemed to be twisting and swirling about the car. My mind had wandered to the scene awaiting our return when my sixteen-year-old's words fell softly upon my ears. "We need a change, Mom. If Dad can't get better, then we need to let him go." The harsh reality of her words chilled us both, yet her wisdom was unquestionable. We had fought this battle long enough.

The statement must have been as difficult for her as his illness had been. Here he was, the good-looking, energetic father, the Air Force pilot, the engineer, the math whiz, the carpenter. His credentials were impressive and the children had been so proud. He always knew the answers no one else did, and as we opened our home and our hearts to our children's friends, he had let them use his computers and helped them build their pinewood derby cars.

Now that person we had all known and loved was gone. He had been lost somewhere, left behind on the battlefield. A new personality had seemed to emerge in his form, a stranger to us. Someone concerned only with his own needs. As understandable as that had been, it was hardest on the children. Friends couldn't come over anymore unless they hid silently away in someone's room or the basement, and loud music was totally out of the question.

Even the television was seldom on. Our four-year-old spent most of his time with the neighbors or relatives, and the wild, fun house had become almost tomb-like, with a shrine of medical paraphernalia and odors incensed with sickness.

How hard it must have been to introduce her dates. And yet she had done it, and still with pride in her voice. Somehow the vision of his former self had continued to shine for her. But now, some crack had appeared in the barrier that she had placed around herself to keep out the truth of his destiny. It was time to open the floodgates and time to let go.

*December 10, 1985*

*Dear Mother,*

*Dad asked about the finances again when I spoke with him on the phone last week. Please, please tell him we will not have to sell our house. I don't know what's going to happen, but it will work out somehow. I was offered a six-week, substitute teaching job, but Dave needs too much care to be left alone. Something will turn up.*

*What upsets me the most is that his death will take care of these problems. I want him to keep going as long as he wants to, but I see the bank account quickly diminishing. Dave keeps asking how the money's holding out, and I keep saying, "Okay. We're good for another two months," or, "Until Christmas." Something like that.*

*Too much to worry about. I'm really tired tonight. Ryan's been sick again with a fever and I have to keep him separated from Dave. It hasn't been a great week.*

*Something fantastic did happen, though. The door bell rang last night, and when I got to the door no one* *was there, but on the porch was a 20-pound turkey with a $100 bill taped to its breast! I couldn't believe it! Last week I got a note in the mail with another $100 bill. Santa came early. I guess it's going to be Christmas after all.*

*Much love,*

*Kathleen*

It was a cold, windy day, and as I drove along, out of the corner of my eye I could see Dave hunched over in the seat beside me. He was always cold now, and I had put him in long underwear that morning. But even the extra layer had not stopped the shivers. To keep him warm I had tucked a large, fluffy quilt around him and under his legs. As the car wove along the twisting road that took us to the highway he swayed back and forth, leaning against the car's direction to offset the movement that was throwing him about. The problem was that when the car turned his reflexes weren't fast enough to correct, and so in his mass of blanket he bobbled this way and that like a first-time rider on a galloping horse.

At the hospital's entrance he asked me, for the first time, to bring a wheelchair out to the car. I pushed him in, parking him out of the door's draft while I moved the car, and then came back. As I approached him he looked like a little old man, and it broke my heart that we had come to this.

Before we saw the doctor we headed in for the routine blood test. His veins were so weak now from the chemo treatments that even the experts had trouble drawing his blood. They tried vein after vein as I stood by watching, wanting to help in some way, to reach out and absorb some of the pain myself. His hunched-over frame rested lightly on the stool as he joked with the technicians. We were regulars these days, and I knew them all well enough to notice when one had changed her hairstyle or was wearing new shoes. As they searched for a vein after tightening the strip of rubber hose around his upper arm, he raised his head slightly, eyes closed, and held his breath. Then the prick came, the needle entering his dried-out, leathery skin searching for a vein whose walls would be strong enough to withstand the puncture before collapsing. Sometimes they would try again and again and then the other arm. It was an ordeal he could never get used to. He had dreaded it every time over the long months and was always exhausted with relief when it was over. Finally success, and enough blood found its way into the vial.

The visit with the doctor was brief, and on the way out Dave had to use the restroom. I helped him into the tiny cubicle and then waited outside by the wheelchair. I busied myself reading an article posted on a nearby bulletin board about the proper technique for a self breast exam. After quite some time had passed, I called to him, offering help. Perhaps forgetting where we were, he lashed back with a sharp, "Leave me alone! I don't need your help!" It caught me at one of those open moments and the words pierced my facade of control leaving a gaping hole. I hoped no one else had heard, and turned around, teary-eyed, only to meet the gaze of the two oncology nurses, who were huddled in conversation watching me. I burst into sobs and started past them, wanting to flee out the door. They stretched out their arms as I came near, and we stood in the hallway in a group hug as they patted me reassuringly on the back. "Don't give in now," they urged. "You've done a great job here, and it's not the time to let it get the best of you. We are so proud of you. There are so many patients who come here alone because no one will come with them."

**David Nielson**
55-65-01/5

## STAFF NOTES

1/3/86    Mr. Nielson is a
gentleman with pancreatic
CA who returns one
month after his last clinic
visit. Since he was last
seen the patient has
required less. . . . His
appetite continues to
remain poor as well, and
he has lost 4 1/4 pounds
since his clinic visit one
month ago.

1/10/86   David had a follow-up CT
scan performed this past
Friday, which initially was
interpreted as showing no
change in tumor size. On
the final written report,
however, new areas of
disease were noted to
have been seen outside
the primary pancreas
tumor mass on further
review. . . .

**PHYSICAL EXAMINATION**: He is somewhat sedated and chronically ill-appearing. His blood. . . .

**IMPRESSION**: Progressive pancreatic cancer outside the primary tumor involving inguinal nodes. . . .

**PLAN**: The patient's radiation will be stopped, he will be treated for his hypercalcemia with prednisone and mithramycin, and the question of reinstitution of FAM will be reviewed next week.

Putting the Cheerios back into the cupboard on Thursday morning, I realized that the doctor had not called me with the results of the blood test. He had always called before. Knowing it was his day in the research lab, I summoned him there. His secretary answered and put me right through.

"I'm sorry," he said. "I just couldn't do it yet. I was going to call this afternoon."

"What do you mean?"

"Well, you must have noticed that things are not a lot better than they were before the treatment last Friday."

"Yes, but what exactly does that mean? This has been up and down for a long time."

"It's only going to be a few more days, Kathleen."

"Days? Days? What happened to the months?"

"I'm sorry." And then my mind, blurred and numb, registered the technical information it already knew but had rejected. All of the symptoms and signs he mentioned I had seen, and, true enough, I had known for some time that it would be the calcium buildup. Somehow I had been caught not looking.

"What will it be like?"

"It will be quiet. He will go to sleep. There will most likely be a coma first. Do you want to tell him?"

"Should I? I don't think I want to."

Carefully, he said, "I think it would be a good decision if you don't want to. You know he'll want to come back to the hospital and get treatment. That could only prolong things for a week or two and it would be awfully hard."

"Can I keep him at home?"

"Yes, I think you can. If it becomes too much you can call Hospice or have him come to the hospital and we'll make him comfortable but give no life support."

"Thank you," I mumbled.

"Call if you need to."

"Good-bye."

My feet were so heavy I had to drag myself up the stairs. Dave was still asleep in our bed and I needed to see him, to sit beside him. The slight jostling of the bed caused him to open his eyes, and he asked, "Is today the day we go to the doctor?"

"No, tomorrow," I answered.

"Good. I don't feel like going anywhere. I think I'll just sleep. Maybe I'll be stronger then."

It's true, I thought. He really is fading. My mind raced. What is the proper procedure here? What preparations do I make? How do I help him get ready?

"I'm going to run a shower for you, Dave. Brent is coming over in a few minutes."

I took a folding chair and set it up in the shower with a towel over it. Then I turned on the water and went to undress him. This morning he was too weak to do much of anything. I wondered if this were a good idea, but he needed a shower and it would make him feel better, so while I tugged and he leaned we got him into position. It actually worked out pretty well until the hairwashing. I had on a pair of sweats that were, by then, soaking and had been keeping him upright in the chair because he didn't seem to have the strength to support himself. I had to release my grip on him to reach the shampoo, and as I did he lost consciousness. I was able to keep him on the chair, but I had to hold onto him with both hands, so I leaned my head back until it hit the water faucet and with a couple of hard taps succeeded in shutting it off. I managed to grab the towel hanging over the door with my teeth and drape it over his shoulders. I didn't know what to do next.

The doorbell rang and I remembered that Brent was coming over. I was afraid he would leave when I didn't answer. I just stood there, soaking wet, covering Dave's ears with the towel, screaming, "Come in!" All at once he was at the bathroom door. Still in his winter coat, he rescued us.

*Did you tackle that trouble that came
your way*
   *With a resolute heart and cheerful?*
*Or hide your face from the light of day*
   *With a craven soul and fearful?*
*Oh, a trouble's a ton, or a trouble's an
ounce,*
   *Or a trouble is what you make it.*
*And it isn't the fact that you're hurt
that counts,*
   *But only how did you take it?*

I can hear her thin, soft voice through the crack of the door. "Do you think it would be okay," she had asked, "if I read to Dad? I mean do you think he might hear me or know I'm there?"

"Of course he'll know," I had answered her, not really believing it. But hadn't I read somewhere that the sense of hearing is often still acute in a comatose person? Perhaps he *can* hear her.

*You are beaten to earth? Well, well,
what's that?*
   *Come up with a smiling face.*
*It's nothing against you to fall down flat,*
   *But to lie there — that's disgrace.*

*The harder you're thrown, why the*
*higher you bounce;*
  *Be proud of your blackened eye!*
*It isn't the fact that you're licked that*
*counts;*
  *It's how did you fight and why?*

I sat down on a chair in the kitchen and strained to hear the melodic sound of her voice as it quietly sang to him the lines of verse. His dear, sweet Kristen. He had loved her so. She had captured that special part of his heart that daddies save for their little girls, and the two of them had a special closeness I had never penetrated. She was his rising star, and he her knight in shining armor. Now she was bidding him farewell.

*And though you be done to death, what*
*then?*
  *If you battled the best you could;*
*If you played your part in the world of*
*men,*
  *Why the Critic will call it good.*
*Death comes with a crawl, or comes with*
*a pounce,*
  *And whether he's slow or spry,*

*It isn't the fact that you're dead that counts,*
  *But only, how did you die?*
                  *Edmund Vance Cooke*

As the glass door of the church slowly closed behind me, I found myself standing alone in the warmth of a January thaw. It had been a gray, overcast week, but this Sunday had dawned bright and clear. As I stepped down the sidewalk in my rush to the car I raised my face to the sky and said aloud, "Please, God, don't let him die on a cloudy day."

The ride home is about five minutes long, but as I started up the hill near our house it stretched to cover the days of our life that we had spent walking through the hills and valleys of our neighborhood to the base of the nearby mountains. We had weaved through the oak brush, jumping across the rushing streams that furrow their way through the foothills, and had watched the seasons come and go. These were the times I had loved best. I had had his undivided attention and we would plan and discuss the children, ourselves, and the future.

As I crested the hill, I was touched by the sudden realization that we would never again hear together the early morning pheasant calls or scare up deer together in the brush. Tears started down my cheeks, and I felt the weight in my chest begin to expand. With only a block and a half to go, I pushed away the pain of what was happening and wiped away the tears.

As I entered the driveway, my brother who had come to be with us for a few days, came out of the house toward the car. Again I was impressed with the warmth of the day, as he appeared quite comfortable in shirtsleeves. Only then did the peculiarity of his coming outside begin to register. I jumped from the car knowing why he was greeting me, but pushing it back . . . not yet . . . not yet. . . .

"What is it?" I asked.

"It's over." He held out his arms to me.

"How do you know?" I could hear my voice saying. Inside I was shouting: He doesn't know! He really doesn't know! He's not a doctor! How can he know? We need to do something! It's not time yet!

"I know," he answered softly.

For a frozen moment I thought I should cry, scream, do something. Then it was gone. Dave's existence was over. All I could say was, "Can I see him? Should I?"

"It will be okay," he said.

I had witnessed scenes such as this in books and movies. I had actually mentally rehearsed how I would behave. Now I was on stage and as I entered the room where he lay I forgot my lines. There was no script. I stood in the doorway for a brief moment and gazed at the body in the bed where I had left Dave only an hour before. The room had not changed in appearance and still carried the familiar "sick" odor that had become part of our existence; but the thin pale shape in the bed was somehow foreign to me. It was no longer my husband. I felt obligated to touch almost out of curiosity. Yes, the cheek was cool and almost solid to the touch. Something inside of me said, "Now you're supposed to bend over and kiss him." I didn't want to. Dave was gone. He wasn't in the bed anymore. Somehow he had left this shell, this covering, and he was somewhere else. The tears still weren't coming and I wondered if I was playing this all wrong. Then I realized that I wasn't the only player. The principal character was not visibly present but was creating an impact nevertheless.

I didn't think of it as relief, but only as peace. I was surely not relieved that my husband was dead, that I was a widow, that my children were fatherless, that for the first time in my life I was the bottom line. But a peace surrounded me that only comes when things are in order, like a job well done. The dishes are washed, the house is clean, you've just put away the last of the folded laundry, and the children are all in bed.

*May it comfort you to know*

*how much he meant*

*to so many.*

*We have all lost someone*

*very special.*

Brent and Pam Nielsen

We had all known it was coming, and yet the shock of death itself seemed so wrong, so out of step. We had grown accustomed to the illness and its trauma. Even the last few days when he'd been comatose had seemed somewhat normal for us. And yet how different that was from the actual fact that he was gone, dead.

Almost instantaneously a numbness had overcome me. It was in some ways like the beginning, all over again. As his diagnosis had heralded a call to far and near, news of his death was quickly whispered about the neighborhood and circulated rapidly among our friends. Food was brought in and the phone was in constant use.

After calling the mortuary I went back in to see Dave. Someone had removed the bottles of medicine from the nightstand and straightened the bed covers. I sat down in the chair beside the bed and tried to figure out what I was feeling. I seemed so void of emotion. I had closed the door and could hear people on the other side of it coming into the kitchen. Their voices were hushed. I supposed they imagined me weeping or holding his hand, but instead I had been wishing they would all leave and I could just curl up in the chair beside his bed and sleep for a while. My legs and arms seemed so heavy I didn't even want to move.

I just sat there as the afternoon sun reflected off the snow outside and shone brightly through the window. Someone had rolled a towel up and put it under Dave's chin to hold his mouth closed. That had been the most distracting thing about his lifeless body. I had wanted to close his mouth myself, but when I had applied pressure in hopes of bringing his chapped, flaking lips together, the rigid muscles had opposed me. I had been unsuccessful. Now, someone who knew more than I had been able to adjust his mouth into a more comfortable-looking and relaxed position.

I sat there alone with his body, curiously scrutinizing its form. The murmurings on the kitchen side of the door faded from my mind and only occasionally did I turn away my intended gaze, realizing that the fine-tuned sound waves were signs of life. Living, breathing people. And as I sat, an aura of peace surrounded me. Like a delicate mist it rose, encircled me, and cloaked itself about my tired body. Peace, as soft and warm as my favorite blanket.

This tranquil sensation was in such contrast to the emotions I had experienced the day before. His stiff comatose body had responded with deep groans of protest as we moved him from side to side to change the bed. Until then I hadn't known that someone in his state of unconsciousness could react verbally to pain. I had felt so trapped knowing that he had to be moved, and yet wanting so desperately for him to be at peace his last few days.

So now there I was, sitting beside his body noticing that it still bore a tense, pained expression. I had thought death brought peace to the physical body as well. Or maybe that is the mortician's job. Is peace of death brought only to the soul that has been allowed to escape its mortal toil? Oh, how I myself wanted to join him and step ahead still holding his hand, still strengthened by sharing my load with him.

Shuddering at the impropriety of such a step and setting my mind toward the next few days, I wondered why I felt such a disassociation from his body. It seemed so void of him, like clothes he had worn out and tossed aside as if they didn't fit anymore. He now had dressed for a new position, a new station in life. Maybe that is what it's like, and here I was left again with the clean-up detail. I knew I could do it. I knew that I would do it no matter how much I wanted to run away. But I wanted a sign. Just some kind of verification that life would go on for me, and that all would be well here. I did have the feeling, this settling peacefulness, but I knew it wouldn't last forever. Feelings never stay the same. I wanted something concrete to hold on to.

I thought of the people I knew who said they'd heard voices. I concentrated, opening up my mind, deeply desiring to hear some murmur of comfort. Nothing. No lightning flashes, no rumbles of thunder. Nothing. But there was still the calmness, the absence of pain, the release of a spirit that had been trapped and tormented for eight long months. Perhaps the voice I had wanted to hear was quietly speaking.

From outside a car's racing engine caught my attention, and when the vehicle's door clapped shut I knew they had come for him. It was so sad to think of his leaving the house for good, the house we had built together, the house I would still be living in.

Quietly, I entered the kitchen as someone else answered the door. Two men with a portable stretcher and a black vinyl bag were the new arrivals. It had not occurred to me that he would leave in a bag, and a suffocating wave of protest rose and then subsided. I hated the thought.

To cover my resistance I began asking questions. "Could you make him fuller faced?"

"Yes." I gave them a picture.

"You must realize, though, he won't look quite this good."

I nearly laughed out loud at the absurdity of the thought.

"Okay," I said. "Just do your best, and I have one last request. I don't want to see him leave, so I will go outside until you've gone if there aren't any more questions."

I stood in the backyard welcoming the warmth of the sun on my face and trying not to visualize their procedure. I paced the length of the patio and made idle conversation with a couple of friends until once again I heard the racing engine. As the gritty crunch of tires on sandy pavement met my ears, I was reaching for the kitchen door.

Back inside I discovered myself in the midst of a great many people. I had thought I wanted to be alone, but the aura of love and concern emanating from their presence was a welcome embrace.

Many of our friends and neighbors who had known the end was near must have started cooking when they were warned, for the house had suddenly filled with mountains of good food. Looking around at the people and the food I pictured one of our many parties, but the thought quickly vanished when I saw his bedclothes carried to the laundry room. I saw the bearer put them in the washer and a wave of gratitude swept over me as I realized I would not have to do this final cleanup. Feeling thirsty, I turned to open the refrigerator, and as I did the sight of its shiny, clean sides and glistening shelves shocked me. What had happened to the splashes of jam, the dried-on juice, and the curled-up carrots?

"We hope you don't mind," the unsolicited helper whispered in my ear. "We wanted so badly to do something."

So there it was. No matter what numbness I felt, no matter how much emotional pain I had suffered, there were still things to do. Things, trivialities I would have to do. I suspected they would get easier as time passed on, but for the moment I wasn't alone and I alone would not have to do them all.

*January 20, 1986*

*Dear Kathleen and Kids,*
*Our hearts go out to you at this time. We wish we could help the pain go away. Just remember you have friends who care. God Bless You.*

*Frank, JoAnn, & boys*

# OBITUARY

SANDY, David R. Nielson, age 43. Died Sunday, January 19, 1986, at home, of pancreatic cancer.

Born June 28, 1942, to Eugene and Eudora Nielson. Raised in Ephraim, Utah; graduated from Manti High School, 1960; graduated University of Utah, 1964; BSEE. He worked for U.S. Steel in Walnut Creek, CA, 1964-65; served an LDS Mission, Great Lakes area, 1965-67; attended Brigham Young University, 1967-68. Married Kathleen Vaughn in the Manti Temple, June 27, 1968.

During the Vietnam era he served five years in the Air Force and was a KC135 pilot. He returned to the Salt Lake Valley where he was employed by various electronics firms before establishing his own consulting business. During his career he designed such various electronic equipment as navigation systems for E-Systems, medical electronics for Bunnell, Inc., and a PROM programmer for Dynatec Intl. He spent his last five years doing what he enjoyed most, designing electronics as a free-lance consultant.

He and his wife built their own home; he was an avid tennis player, loved the outdoors, was active in Cub Scouting, and collecting and restoring antiques. Dave's fellow professionals have great respect for his ability as an electronics designer and engineer. Among his many friends, relatives, and neighbors he had the well deserved reputation of being able and willing to fix any household item from sprinkler systems to broken furniture. He was dearly loved and will be greatly missed.

He is survived by his wife; his daughter Kristen, age 16; and his sons, Scott, 14, and Ryan, 4; Mother, Eudora Nielson, Ephraim; Brothers, Gerald E., Jay C., Salt Lake City; Sisters, Carol Orgil, Richland, WA, and Lorraine Ross, Cedar City, Utah.

I sighed with relief as I noticed the strain had been removed from his furrowed brow. His face, not as full as at healthy times, had lost its gaunt, bony appearance, and his body, clothed in the temple robes of our church, seemed finally at peace. I stood back and looked at the humble casket. I knew there were some who would not approve, but Dave would have.

Ever since our marriage, he'd expressed fears of his death and my being taken advantage of through the high cost of dying. He had always given me rambling lectures on how poor widows were robbed of their last penny by money-hungry undertakers. My experience with the mortuary had not been representative of Dave's views, but perhaps it had been easier because the choices had already been made.

Just eight days earlier I had brought up the subject of an actual funeral for the first time. The January sun had been pouring in the family room's east windows all morning and its heat had filled the room, contrasting with the snow and cold outside. Dave had spent an hour sitting on the sofa talking to a business associate about the work he was going to do as soon as he was well enough. I had looked over from my kitchen duties to see his delicate frame still spontaneous, still enthusiastic, responding to the plans being offered him. I knew it must be terribly difficult because earlier that morning I had finally said what I had been thinking for a long time. "If there's good time left, Dave, you've got to give some of it to your family." He had agreed that he had selfishly put all of his good moments and thoughts toward his work. So he was trying to step back, step down, and let go of it.

After the associate left I had gone over to sit with him. We had spoken about the snow, the doctor's appointment the day before when he'd received a treatment for his high calcium blood level, and what the agenda was for the next week. Then as casually as I could I had said, "By the way, if I'm killed in a car wreck or something happens to me, please make sure that Patti sings at the funeral, and that no one preaches too much."

"Consider it done," he responded and offered nothing more.

I knew he hadn't wanted to talk about it, but he wasn't the only one involved here. I had gone on, "So tell me Dave, is there anything you would or would not want me to do if I had to do a funeral for you?"

"Nope, you can do anything you want, just don't spend a lot of money."

Gingerly, I took it one step further. "Is there anyone you might like to have speak that was from your life before you met me?"

After pondering for a moment he slowly shook his head and answered, "No, Kathleen, my life started when I met you."

In one quick instant I both loved and hated him for saying it. For nearly eight long months he'd been pushing against death's door, and yet never once had anything personal crossed his lips. I had tried to do everything for him. I had bathed, fed, dressed, cleaned up after, and nursed him. Throughout that time he had not been able to tell me of his love. He had never been a verbal person, and all of our married life I had longed to hear endearments. Now, as he was about to leave me behind, he had given me the ultimate compliment, and I had only looked at him, not knowing what to say.

The doorbell had then rung, breaking into our tender moment. His friend Brent had come to sit with him while I ran an errand. My errand had taken me to the place where I was now standing, the mortuary near our home. I smiled, remembering how I had told the funeral director, "I don't want any surprises. I need to know what funerals cost." I had explained that I was anticipating a death about two months down the road and I needed to know the facts before I had to make the decisions. Upon my request he had dropped the low-voiced, over-compassionate approach, and we had gotten along well. By the time I left I had toured the facility, been briefed on how to write an obituary, and understood how easily I could spend a great deal of money.

On the way home I had remembered how Dave, when first ill, had spoken of making a wooden casket to save money. At that time thoughts of death had been such a mystery. He had said he and Scott could build one and we could keep it downstairs. Quickly I had come back with, "No! Absolutely not! No one here is going to make their own casket and let it sit around waiting!" That had been the last discussion about anything to do with funerals.

When I got home Brent was ready to leave. I walked him out to the car and offered him a special proposal.

"You may think this is crazy," I said. "But what would you say about making a wooden casket for Dave? No, don't respond now, and you won't have to do the inside, but think about it and call me."

The phone rang an hour later. "First of all," Brent said, "There are people who won't like this, Kathleen. They'll think it's weird, or crazy, or just not right. But I think it's great. How much time do we have?"

"On Friday the doctor said about two months," I told him.

An hour later the phone rang again. "This is going to be great," he said again. "Do you want brass handles or wooden handles, and the dimensions just have to fit the vault. Right?"

"Listen," I said. "Just let me know the details when you have it figured out. Okay?"

I had turned away from the phone wanting to run and tell Dave of our plans. I hadn't. Sometime in the next two months, I thought.

# S E R V I C E S
*Wednesday, January 22, 1986 - 1:00 p.m.*
*Bishop John L. Riley, Conducting*

FAMILY PRAYER . . . . . . . . . . . . . . . Jay C. Nielson
PRELUDE-POSTLUDE MUSIC . . . . . . . . Pam Nielsen
INVOCATION . . . . . . . . . . . . . . . . . Jon Young
REMARKS . . . . . . . . . . . . . . . . . Eric Nielson
MUSICAL SELECTION . . . . . . . . . . . . . "The Rose"
*Patti Maxfield, accompanied by James Prigmore*
REMARKS . . . . . . . . . . . . . . . . Michael Guarino
REMARKS . . . . . . . . . . . . . Bishop John L. Riley
MUSICAL SELECTION . . . . . . . . . "Through the Years"
*Patti Maxfield, accompanied by James Prigmore*
BENEDICTION . . . . . . . . . . . . . . David B. Vaughn

\*

## GRAVESIDE SERVICES

Taps . . . . . . . . . . . . . . . . . . . . . . Jeff Grundvig
*Folding of the Colors*
*Larry Vaughn, Scott Nielson, Keith Vaughn*

Dedication of the Grave . . . . . . . . . .Gerald E. Nielson

\*

## CASKET LOVINGLY CRAFTED BY:
Scott and Kristen Nielson,
Doug and Carla Johnson,
Brent and Pam Nielsen,
Charles and LaRae Wilson,
Joe and Cheryl Gale,
Lee and Chris Skidmore,
Jeremy and Jennifer Nielsen,
Tim and Elaine Larson.

Standing beside the casket, I can see the line of people waiting to speak with me getting longer. I'm glad I put out the photo albums and displayed the collected mementos of his life's time and accomplishments. I can see people looking at them and I think of how only a few minutes ago Janice, from Cleveland, was showing Charlotte the photos taken when we lived as neighbors in Indiana.

Hanging on display, Dave's flat tweed cap, a gift from his brother to cover his smooth, hairless head over the past months, has brought tears to several eyes. His patent, a PROM programmer circuit board, and his tennis racket all evoke some memory for each of us.

Standing here beside his body, now merely a representation of him, I am strengthened by the love of our family and friends. Somehow in all of this pain there seems to be an order in what's happening, like an eternal fitness of things. If only we could see beyond the veil that keeps us separated from those who've gone on. Dave's presence has been so strong these last few days that I could swear he's been beside me at times. I've even worried about it a little. But will I always *want* his presence felt?

What was that? The short stocky man who just came through the line, someone I've never seen before. He must have worked with Dave somewhere. He just leaned toward me and whispered in my ear, "I just want you to know that it's okay to go on. I lost my wife some time ago and married a widow. Sometimes we feel her husband's influence, and sometimes we feel my wife's, and it's okay. I just want you to know that when this is all over it will be okay to go on." Looking out into the main group of people, I can't see him now. Who was he?

Sometimes as I look out at those here I only see past them and take in the sprays of flowers that are everywhere. I never knew they could mean so much. Dave's probably stewing a little over their expense, but since they all come from friends I can simply enjoy them.

Just moments ago I was concerned that the children were destroying the beautiful gold mums by the head of the casket. There's a door right behind the flowers there, and it has been opening and closing all night as the children have brought people there to see where they and the other casket makers have engraved their names in the soft pine of their father's coffin.

It had been such a turnaround for them to be able to participate in the making of it. Scott at first had been reluctant and Kristen enthusiastic. In the end they had both gone with Brent to the school's hobby shop. It had been a hurried process, and as Dave had slipped slowly into a coma that Friday, Brent, Kristen, and Scott joined by others from our old neighborhood, had proceeded to fulfill my wish of having a special pine box for Dave.

Late that night I had grown concerned and had driven over to the school hobby shop to pick them up. No one had been there. I then had driven to Brent and Pam's house. Walking up to the door I had been shocked to hear laughter. When I had gone in I had found my children free of the heavy, invisible burden they'd carried for the past months. Somehow, physically participating in making a contribution to their father's passing had enabled them to accept it. The laughing had been over the too-short board Brent had cut, the gouge from Scott's hammer miss, and how they had all said that they weren't sure Dave, himself, hadn't been there bossing the job, telling Kristen to clean up the glue joints and Pam to get more nails – familiar tunes that over the years he had helpfully whistled at all of us.

*January 21, 1986*

*Dear Kathleen,*

*We found and all signed this card, but we all felt that some important things were left unsaid; foremost, what this experience of working on the casket has meant to us. For us all the initial idea was startling as I'm sure it is for most, but as we began planning and eventually working, we all were deeply touched by our involvement. In these situations we all long to have any opportunity of helping, but are basically unable to do much to really reduce suffering or to contribute anything really significant. In this case we all feel the reward of doing something that did matter. Your idea not only fulfilled your and Dave's wishes, but allowed your friends to participate in a true labor of love. From everyone who sanded, nailed, measured, and stained, thank you for this gift which we now, completed, return to you.*

Remembering the funeral, I hear the pleading voice of Ryan, my four-year-old, as he called out through the fraction of time that would have otherwise been silent. Questioning, wondering, and stating the desire of all our hearts.

This thing, this ominous darkness that had come into our lives. How did it happen? Why did the scourge stop at our door? Is there a reason? Is there an explanation for the pain inflicted upon our family? Were we singled out? Did we need to be taught something? Was it simply the luck of the draw?

Our lives were so full. The long-worked-for successes were adding up, and a contentment that seems to come to only a few had settled itself around our home. Then suddenly a knife, unsheathed, struck through the brightness of our day and pierced our shield of armor to our core. It twisted and gouged our innermost selves, tearing at our very existence. The pain was incredible and throbbed throughout every moment of our day. It became a nightmare shrieking with horror and destruction, but we never woke up. The minutes became hours, and then the hours became minutes as we realized that even nightmares have an end, and the finish to this one would leave such a void that we would cling at whatever cost to what we knew and loved.

But somewhere along the way the cost became too great. The torture, the suffering itself, began demanding a toll that seemed insupportable. The very expression of hope drained itself from our thoughts and a waiting game was played. Some moves were longer than others, and some had greater rewards than the next, but they were all plotted in one direction and at times the goal seemed unbelievably close.

The only escape was to remember happier times. The six-thousand-mile car trip to Vermont. Three kids and two adults in a van for twenty-two days of vacation. What a miracle that had been. We had no car trouble, no one fought too memorably, and no one got sick. And the days in the Air Force, moving around the country, flying around the world, and being taken care of by Uncle Sam. Then there was building our own house, becoming self-employed, and looking forward to a future that seemed to offer everything we'd ever dreamed of. A future that we were now being robbed of.

How we longed for the life we had before the termination order came. How we would give all the worldly possessions back for another chance.

Oh, how my four-year-old's words come hauntingly back to me. We were on the front pew in the chapel and the pine box in front of us was close enough to touch. As his words, simple and innocent, were heard, a wave of love and tears rippled through the congregation. The pleading words of a four-year-old, "I want my Daddy back."

*January 28, 1986*
*Journal entry*

*Kathryn Mehr called me this morning.*
*She said the astronauts were in the*
*water, that the shuttle launch had*
*malfunctioned. I turned on the*
*television to watch. Later when Kristen*
*came home from school she looked at*
*me and said, "I know who will be*
*debriefing them, Mom."*

She must think I'm crazy. My poor, sweet neighbor who came to the rescue without so much as a question. Am I going to need people forever? Surely this state of dysfunction won't last.

I could never have made it through the eight months of Dave's illness without them, however, and the help they offered. The notes from friends and neighbors that I would find in the mailbox. "We didn't want to bother you, but we wanted you to know we care, we're thinking about you, and we want to help if there's anything at all we can do." The people who showed up at the hospital time and time again as we returned time and time again. Sondra, nurse and neighbor, who came at a moment's call to give shots or usher us to the hospital. The food that was consistently delivered, and the gracious neighbors who absorbed Ryan into their lives. Charlotte, the friend who stood by my side and was able to arrange her schedule to ours as she accompanied me to and from airports, through doctors' evaluations, and had taken notes so efficiently at the mortuary as we made the final arrangements. Mike, the family friend who had rubbed my feet when they ached, tutored Kristen in trigonometry until 2 a.m., wrestled with Ryan from one end of the family room to the other, and counseled Scott in what they both smilingly said was, "Proper male behavior with the opposite sex."

All of the friends, all of the caring had been a Godsend.

Now the crisis is over. Dave is laid to rest. Kristen and Scott are in school full time. Ryan watches "Sesame Street" and plays with the neighborhood children. I wander around the house listening to the quiet, or sit in the family room staring out the window. My main job has been terminated. The frenzy and rush of my days have disappeared overnight. Only a few people call now, and I wonder how much of me has died with Dave. I just want to sleep, but sleep won't come.

I had thought that his death would bring relief. Instead it has brought disorientation. I am lost. The trail isn't clearly marked anymore. I need a line to follow, or at the very least a vague direction.

It's like I'm standing in this huge candy store of life. One minute I want to taste everything in sight. The next minute I want a piece of the green peppermint. No, the chocolate peanut cluster. No, the sugary lemon drops. Then I quietly leave empty-handed, thinking nothing would have tasted good anyway.

Why are the choices so hard? Why are the decisions so weighty? Why can't I get moving?

Here I am, totally okay, and yet this morning I wasn't able to do the laundry. It seems so stupid. We have all been out of clean underwear for at least two days, and I've promised each day to do the wash. Then I forget. This morning when I started for the laundry room I thought I would do it. Instead I called Sondra. "I need you to go shopping with me," I said. "If I don't go buy some underwear I'm going to have to do the laundry, and I just can't face doing it."

She didn't even ask why. Somehow she understood my distress. She just came over and we went shopping.

*March 11, 1986*

*Dear Kristen, Scott, and Ryan,*

*I know that sometimes life seems totally empty and without hope. I suspect that you feel like you will never be truly alive again.*

*Carl, a man that worked for my father for eight years, spoke at my father's funeral. He told us kids to talk about our father. We followed that advice, and found that sometimes it made us cry, sometimes laugh, and often we felt proud. It also helped us adjust to the loss.*

*I hope that when your mom cooks something on the stove that your Dad liked, you'll say, "Dad sure loved Mom to make this." Or if it is something he didn't care for, say, "Dad was glad he didn't have to eat this very often."*

*When someone tells you one of those engineering-type mathematical jokes, you can say, "That was Dad's kind of joke. He'd enjoy that."*

*I'm not sure why, but I know if you do talk about Dave that life will start taking meaning more quickly.*

*And I know that is what your father would want.*

*From the hand and heart of somebody you never had to call Mister.*

*Jon, the Rock Man*

*P.S. Ask about the turkeys and I'll tell you a story your dad would enjoy.*

Kneeling on the grave I feel the sharp chill of the metal as my fingers trace the letters of his name, and I wonder why. Not, why me? But, why him? I had prayed a hundred times for the answer. He was strong, capable, productive, and we all loved him so much. Why would he be taken? Why was it allowed to happen? I look to the sky and wonder if there could possibly be meaning to all of this.

I pray for understanding and no answers come. I ask why? How could this be? And I hear only an echo. The echo rings in my brain and reverberates throughout my body. It gains intensity as it resounds and builds to the crescendo of a full symphony before it gradually plays itself out. Weakened, I raise my head and wonder how much strength is left. When will the answers come?

If only there could be a tangible explanation. Something concrete to visualize. How could a normal, healthy man be stricken with such a vengeance; torn, twisted, mutilated, and then discarded, thrown aside? No one can tell me. And now even God, Himself, is holding back.

I am uncertain of what lessons are supposed to be learned here. If this earth is a trial ground, a place to prove ourselves, then let this be enough. I have done my time. But all my pleading gets me nowhere, and the questions are still unanswered. The wound is fresh and bleeding and I wonder if it will ever heal.

I see others who have suffered as I, and they have gone on with new lives. Do they have more understanding? Are answers available to some? I have seen a few, too, who can't get beyond the pain. How much should we hang on to? Is the folly of those who don't go on, that the pain itself is comforting? Because it's what they know, do they cling to it? Is it harder to let go and move on? Questions, questions, and no easy answers.

With all my energy I resent what's come my way. I think it would be so much easier if there were someone to blame, someone on whom to vent my anger. Someone to have to forgive. There is no one.

So I turn to a higher source and pray for understanding, and the understanding comes too slowly. I find myself questioning my purpose, my being, and wonder if some master plan is at work. Are we merely stringed puppets on a stage, being jerked and pulled this way and that? At times I feel as though I have been danced to the edge of a precipice and teeter there unsure of my footing. I find myself wanting to jump, hoping my strings will be severed and I will float through space until I've been swallowed up by the distance. Other times I want to wrap the strings about me to insure my safekeeping.

I remember the day I drove through a low cloud that had settled itself on the foothills near my home. I was submerged in grayish white light and felt confused, disoriented, and helpless. But as I passed beyond the cloud and emerged once again into the clear light of day, I was filled with reassurance of a future. At the time I had wondered if maybe that was what was happening to my life. I had been going along enjoying the view, when suddenly a cloud had appeared. A fog that's denseness had seemed immeasurable. A covering that had blocked the light of day. And like the cloud I had driven through and left behind, would I someday be free of this mantle of grief that now weighed me down?

I push this shroud of thoughts from my mind and try to remember how fresh the morning sun feels when it comes over the mountains bringing light again to the valley below. I cling to the hope of that light, knowing that even at the darkest times over the months of illness there had been brief moments when the sun had shone through. A few isolated instants when I had still wanted to run with the wind and dance under the stars.

Maybe there is hope of a good life ahead after all. Maybe it's not important to have all the answers right now. Perhaps with enough time, sunshine, and patience, it will all just fall into place.

*April 4, 1986*

*Dear Kathleen,*

Thoughts of those we care about
Can always make us smile
Because the special times we've
shared
Make life seem more worthwhile . . .
And often on a day like this,
I wonder if you guess
How many times a thought of you
Has brought me happiness!

*Love,*

*Judith*

*I've been thinking about you and the
kids. I hope you are well and
adjusting. I can't believe it has been
three months.*

Will the holidays always be bittersweet? Will they always dredge up pain because Dave is not with us and at the same time evoke sweet memories of those good times we had together?

Mother's Day . . . I had thought we were all okay. With Kristen away at school, Scott, Ryan, and I had driven down to Dave's mother's house for the afternoon. Traditionally that's what we would have done anyway, and it had seemed right. It had been right, and after the fried chicken, cream gravy, and corn fritters we had started the two-hour drive home. Ryan fell asleep immediately in the back seat, and to break the unnatural silence that stretched between Scott and myself, he punched one of our home-recorded cassette tapes into the dashboard player. "Hello darkness my old friend . . . ," Simon and Garfunkel sang from the speakers.

"Take it out!" I blurted while reaching for the volume knob.

Scott blocked my hand and said emphatically, "No! Leave it in."

"I can't hear that right now," I said. "That's your dad's favorite tape. We've listened to that on every car trip we ever made."

"I know," he answered. "Let's keep it on."

"And the vision that was planted in my brain still remains within the sounds of silence."

"I can't, Scott. I just can't. The day, our first time at his house without him, I'll come to pieces."

"Maybe we need to, " he responded.

"Like a bridge over troubled waters, I will ease your mind."

The tears started silently, streaked down my cheeks, and dripped from my chin onto my blouse. I looked over at Scott and his visible pain released a choking sob from my own throat. His whole face was wet. There were big red blotches around his eyes where his clenched fists had been wiping away the salty flow. I wanted to stop the car, embrace him. But silently I turned my attention back to the road, slowing down a little. The car's warmth and solid shell surrounded us in our grief like a cocoon. We were a captive audience to one another's pain as the music poured forth.

"And yes, we've just begun, sharing horizons that are new to us," as the Carpenters took over. With them came the memories of years past. They danced through our minds and filled the spaces around us. The memories tugged and tore at us as the pain went deeper and deeper. "Just like before . . . It's yesterday once more . . . "

For an hour the car rolled along, Ryan slept, and Scott and I continued to purge our innermost selves through tears of anguish, regret, and longing. Eventually the canyon road led into the valley, and the wracking sobs slowly diminished to quiet murmurs of spent turmoil. The lights of the city were starting to come on, and they twinkled and blinked at us as the sun's light faded on the horizon.

The last of the tape began to play Peter, Paul and Mary's soothing strains. "The answer, my friend, is blowin' in the wind. The answer is blowin' in the wind."

*May 15, 1986*

*Dear Kathleen,*

*I just wanted to do something special for you and your family . . . Because I think the world of you all and love you very much.*

*The book* My Gift from Jesus *is for the kids. I cry every time I read it. But it makes things seem clearer even to an old person like me.*

*The frame with the embroidered quote is for you. Consider it a memento from the funeral and the song Patti sang there. "The Rose" is one of my favorite songs. The words, "It's the heart afraid of breaking, that never learns to dance," apply to you and Dave and also to your future, Kathleen.*

*If there's anything you or the kids ever need, please ask.*

*I loved Dave and all of you. You're a very special group of people.*

*I love you all,*

Kola

"**I** know!" I suggested brightly. "Let's go eat our lunch by Daddy's grave." We were driving away from the take-out window of the local fast-food lunch spot, and six-year-old Ryan responded enthusiastically in the affirmative. This procedure had not become a habit with us, but rather an occasional treat. Often we would stay in the car as we divided up the french fries, shared the chicken pieces, or wolfed down the hamburgers. Other times we would sit on the grass near his grave, resting our drinks on the smooth flat headstone. It was a time of reflection and a time to feel close to the memory of Dave. I don't think I've ever felt like he was there, himself, but rather like it is the one place that will remain ours alone. Everything else is changing, and rightfully so. The house is becoming more my home instead of our home, and as the checkbook heading has decreased to one name and the bills now come only to one responsible party, the grave has become the reality of him. At the grave I see his name and remember. There the memories are always good, and Ryan and I talk about his daddy. Pressures to finish the dishes or answer the phone have been left behind. The mountains rise up behind us, their rocky peaks stretching skyward, while the valley lies at our feet with the city poured into its length. In the far west the Great Salt Lake catches and reflects the sun's shimmering rays. Here we have made tracks in fresh snow, seen the crab apple bloom, smelled the petunias, and watched autumn's leaves twirl across the grass.

On this day as our car drew up to its parking spot, Ryan thoughtfully asked, "When will Daddy come back alive? I want him to come back now."

It wasn't the first time he'd asked, and it brought to my mind how simply our innocent children see things. He'd heard the story of the Resurrection at home and at church and remembered that it meant those who die here will have life again. The timetable of childhood did not want to wait. "I want to go be with him," he insisted. I tried to explain how the time was not right and how we had many wonderful things to do here before we could go where he was. It all sounded so simple, even to me. Is it the passions and desires of our hearts that complicate it so much?

Getting out of the car we stepped onto the cool, soft grass. Ryan darted ahead of me and I thought of the first time we'd come here after Dave's death. Ryan, with great agitation and the impatience of a four-year-old, had wanted to lift up the ground and get his daddy out of the box. At the time I'd been horrified, and every time I've thought of his words since, my brain has formed a visual image of what possible state Dave's remains might be in. I dismissed the thought with a shiver and uttered a small prayer of gratitude that this site we pay homage to only houses that temporal state, that covering that served as a temporary residence for his spirit.

Ryan and I lay down on the grass and watched the wispy clouds as they chased across the sky in constant change. Ryan moved over and snuggled into the crook of my arm. I took advantage of the time to recall other trips to the graveside.

The first summer after Dave's death Scott and two of his friends, all fifteen, had been anxious to try driving, as none were old enough yet to get licenses. My new Jeep Cherokee was a prime target, and I had cautiously given in. They had come to the cemetery with us one evening, and as Ryan and I had watched the pinks and purples of the dying sun, they had made the rounds of the grounds in my car.

My car that I had proudly driven to the cemetery after its first washing. It had been a warm, sunny day for February, and I had hurried from the carwash to the graveside, where I had toweled it off as the drops were beginning to freeze. I hadn't even said anything that day, as I sometimes did, speaking to myself or to him out loud. I had just wanted to show him.

There was also the time I had rolled down the window of the car as I drove past on my way to the grocery store. In the direction of his grave I had screamed, "You'd better help me, Dave! I don't like this. You'd better find someone for me here!"

And the time in the spring not too long after his death when I had broken into tears at his graveside, wailing something about how I wished I'd been a better wife. Suddenly I had stopped, and wiping the tears away, had blurted out, "And damn it to Hell, I wish you'd been a better husband!"

This last summer when I got my mountain bike I had ridden it over to the cemetery and back. It had brought physical fitness more strongly back into my life, and with it a renewed sense of well being. Somehow riding it there had enabled me to show him how I'd grown.

Smiling to myself I wondered what Dave thought of all this. It seems unfairly balanced in my opinion, for I believe he knows what he wants to know of our lives here. Like the time Kristen was dressed for the prom and with a huge lump in my throat I said, "Oh, how I wish your dad could see you now."

Without missing a beat she had brightly replied, "Oh, I think he can, don't you?"

Sitting in Scott's plays I had often thought Dave, too, was watching him. And at Christmas time, when the kindergartners had caroled for the parents, I had felt so alone. Looking at the empty chair beside me I had thought it a terrible injustice that Dave had not been there to see Ryan perform.

Then I had been filled with that sense of his presence – that indeed he was there, and yes, he did get to see some of those precious moments.

And of course, there's the time on the four-wheeler when I crashed, or nearly crashed. I had had Ryan in front of me, and as we had started down the steep, rutted road I had lost control, accidentally pushing on the gas instead of the brake. We jerked this way and that as I stretched out my feet to keep us upright, hoping we wouldn't tip over. My mind had raced wildly, trying to determine the best plan of action. Should I grab Ryan and try to bail off? Could we clear the vehicle? Can I get this stopped before we are pitched over the dropoff to the side? I had felt a violent pull on my left leg and, yanking hard, had managed to bring it forward. We had then bumped wildly out of the rut up onto a high bank and had suddenly came to an abrupt stop.

Down the hill ahead of us had been Kristen and Scott, anxiously watching our adventure. To our right was a steep, forty-foot drop to a lower road, and ten feet straight ahead the high bank we were on had dropped away to nothing. My feet were still extended and my hands gripped the handlebars in an iron-clad clench. I couldn't figure out what had happened. I wanted to ask the children if they could tell me how the machine had stopped. I had no recollection of ever applying the brakes. Before the question had left my mouth, however, my attention had been directed to the throb in my left shin. I had never seen a deep wound before, and I couldn't figure out what all that whitish-looking stuff had been coming out of my leg. The brain took over then, and seeing the black tire marks up the back of my leg I had realized that the violent jerk had been the back tire running up my calf. The force had banged my shin down onto the rough footrest, which had gouged a deep hole just below my knee. Turning away, I had reached down with my left hand and had grabbed the opening, closing it as best I could, while hollering at Kristen to go get the Jeep.

An hour later I had been lying on a table in the emergency room of the local hospital, waiting for the plastic surgeon to come. Staring at the ceiling, I had been suddenly filled with the immenseness of the possibilities that could have resulted from our situation. My teeth then had begun to chatter and I had felt incredibly cold. Tears started creeping from the corners of my eyes, dripping ticklishly into my ears. Then quietly and softly a warmth had overcome me. At the same time, a familiar voice, soft and reassuring, had whispered to me. I could never remember if there had actually been words, but I felt Dave had been there. I think he had probably been on the hill with us as well.

So it seems to me that those who have gone beyond this life have some special privileges. We, struggling here in this mortal state, have such a small understanding of the total picture.

Breaking into my thoughts, Ryan suddenly jumped up off the grass and ran over to a plastic windmill on a grave down the hill. I called to him for a race to the car and we headed home.

Driving away I realized that even though our trips to the graveside were becoming less and less frequent, they still offered us a place to review, an opportunity to remember the past and to think about the possibilities of the future.

## Epilogue

Someone asked me the other day if I were still angry with my husband for dying. My first thoughts in response were that I didn't know if I'd ever been angry with him specifically. Pondering the matter, I believe that a good portion of my feelings of anger or resentment have been directed toward life itself. I didn't deserve this bump in the road, this setback that has turned my hair silver and robbed me and my children of the future we'd been promised.

Then I look around and wonder what right I have to feel sorry for myself. What makes me so privileged that I should travel through this life without any severe misfortune? And yet there is a little anger, a little resentment hanging in the closet of my thoughts, reaching out, grabbing me at the most unexpected times. I will walk into a theater with a woman friend or one of my children, and looking around all I can see are couples, couples in love out for an evening, holding hands, whispering to one another, sharing, enjoying, loving, and my heart feels as if I am the only one in the whole world without a mate. I walk into church and sit alone surrounded by happy families, families that appear to have no struggles. They are full, complete, healthy, successful, and have everything.

At these times I have to concentrate on the reality of life. I look at those around me and try to imagine what their lives must really be like. It's not simply a matter of getting the hay baled before it rains or the roof on the house before cold weather, for our lives have become so complex and so busy as modern technology and progressive thoughts have overtaken us. Violent storms that surface from within us have often been brewing for years with shifting winds and highs and lows that have slowly weakened the innermost core. So glancing around I question what winds are blowing here in the lives around me. Lives that seem so perfect, so complete, so together. My resentment and anger then become short-lived, and even though they linger to strike out at me again at some weak moment, I have a better perspective. I suppose, however, that there will always be some frustration because I will never know how it would have been had Dave lived.

So once again I play my mind game of remembering the good times, and often that's difficult. It's been almost three years now since his death, and the eight months of illness are still uppermost in my memory of him. If I truly have anger or resentment, it is mostly directed toward the fact that I retain this memory of the "sick" Dave. I have forgiven him for any inconvenience I suffered during that time, but I didn't like the person he often was throughout those months.

I told someone the other day about his inability to speak to me of his dying, and how we had never terminated with one another. We had never said good-bye. My friend was shocked. "You were robbed," she said. And I believe I was, but at the time I had not understood the importance of it.

I felt that one should be allowed to die in his own way. I thought that allowing Dave to be in control of all aspects of his own death was the most appropriate way to handle it. So when I had asked him to please write a letter to each of the children so that they would know what he'd thought of them and what he'd hoped for them and he had said, "No." I had forgiven him. When I had asked him to tell me about our taxes and how to best approach taking care of them and he had said, "Not now." I had dismissed it. When I had wanted to tell him the end was near and how I would miss him, and the doctor had said, "You know he'll just want to come and have more treatment," I had put it away. I had felt that the patient's wishes were the only ones to be considered. I was wrong.

Not long ago I heard a lecture on having a "good death." Put off at first by the sound of it, I soon began to realize how right it was. It seems almost tragic that the one, truly inevitable thing for each of us, is so botched up sometimes. We go out of our way not to prepare for something that's going to happen whether we want it to or not. People die every day without wills, leaving those behind countless financial and emotional problems to deal with because of it. Who gets the money? Who gets the children? How do we sort it out? Others make little attempt to provide financially for their survivors whether through insurance or simply savings for funeral costs.

And most of us tear through life collecting things, surrounding ourselves with paraphernalia we never wanted, never used, or wore out. In the past while, as I have tried to work toward putting my life in a more organized pattern to relieve my children of ever having to deal with my lack of order, I try to remember the old adage our mothers drummed into us about never going anywhere in ragged underwear for fear we'd somehow be found out. Believe me, if someone had had to step into my home had Dave and I both died, the work they would have faced to sort and organize could only have led to anger and resentment. I had trouble enough myself opening the boxes from Dave's past that had been hauled from one home to another and had been rearranged countless times in our basement. While I in turn have kept every letter ever written to me and every textbook since junior high school, as well as the little white box with blue stars on it that contains cockleburs matted with the black hair of our cocker spaniel that was run over by a car in the spring of 1955.

Resentment and anger toward Dave? No, not really. Resentment and anger toward the hand I've been dealt? Yes, sometimes.

Most often when the car breaks down or when Scott's in a play and I go alone to see him. When Kristen gets straight A's or when Ryan wants to go camping. And I suppose most of all when I reach out in the dark to the empty pillow beside me.

And yet . . . I like who I am now better than who I was before. I have a calmer spirit inside of me. I consider negative thoughts a waste of time and I don't harbor petty grievances. I feel as though I have gained a deeper understanding of what's most important in life, which to me is very simply loving and helping others as we experience the throes of this life on earth. I have continued to wave to the UPS driver who hasn't delivered a package to us since Dave's death. I smile at strangers when I walk by, and I make an effort to contact others who I think might be lonely or in need of help.

I have gained a greater sense of appreciation for my physical surroundings as well. "You don't just go hiking!" a friend once said. "You climb mountains!" Yes, I do. And when I'm on the summit, or when the river hike is over and we've climbed up out of the canyon, I am stronger and I am braver because I have pushed myself and succeeded. Because I have stretched my physical capabilities and at the same time reckoned with both the insignificance and the majesty of a single life in the vastness of our universe.

I like who I am. I am not unhappy. At the same time I am not as fulfilled as I would like to be. I miss being married. I miss every aspect of it, and when my little one prays at night that we will find a new daddy I too hope we will.

If Dave could come back today I would welcome him. But I am not the same person I was and things would have to be different. I don't know why it took me forty years and the death of my husband to find out who I really am. Dave always had such a strong self-image perhaps I borrowed from him. Left alone, I have chosen to swim rather than sink. However, I have not been totally alone, for I have been strengthened by my faith in God whom I speak to daily as I kneel in prayer. Sometimes the words are squeaky as they pour out through my sobs of loneliness, but more often they flow in abundance of thankfulness for the opportunities in life that come my way.

I have friends who know how to pick me up when I fall, family that stands unjudgingly by, parents who think I can do no wrong (heaven forbid the day they're not here), children I dearly love, and a good and faithful dog.

I cannot minimize the value of the strength I have received from those around me. And when the voice inside of me says, "You're doing fine. It's going to be all right." I know that it will all be okay even though no one prepared me for this.

*And God shall wipe away all tears from their eyes; and there shall be no more death, neither sorrow, nor crying, neither shall there be any more pain: for the former things are passed away.*

*Revelation 21:4*